CU00960157

FINDING THE RIGHT WORDS

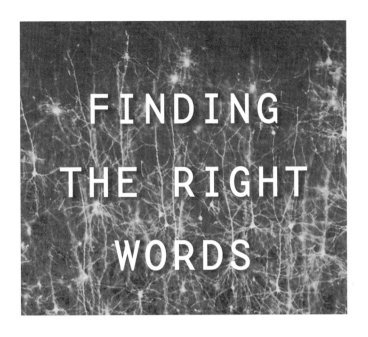

FINDING THE RIGHT WORDS

a story of literature, grief, and
the brain

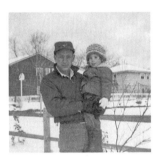

Cindy Weinstein
With **Bruce L. Miller, MD**

Johns Hopkins University Press | BALTIMORE

© 2021 Johns Hopkins University Press
All rights reserved. Published 2021
Printed in the United States of America on acid-free paper
2 4 6 8 9 7 5 3 1

Johns Hopkins University Press
2715 North Charles Street
Baltimore, Maryland 21218-4363
www.press.jhu.edu

Library of Congress Cataloging-in-Publication Data

Names: Weinstein, Cindy, author. | Miller, Bruce L., 1949– author.
Title: Finding the right words : a story of literature, grief, and the brain /
Cindy Weinstein, with Bruce L. Miller, MD.
Description: Baltimore : Johns Hopkins University Press, 2021. |
Includes bibliographical references and index.
Identifiers: LCCN 2020036271 | ISBN 9781421441269 (hardcover) |
ISBN 9781421441276 (ebook)
Subjects: LCSH: Alzheimer's disease—Patients—Biography. |
Parent and child—Relationship
Classification: LCC RC523.2 .W44 2021 | DDC 616.8/3110092 [B]—dc23
LC record available at https://lccn.loc.gov/2020036271

A catalog record for this book is available from the British Library.

Title page images: Layer 5 pyramidal neurons of the human cerebral
cortex stained using the rapid Golgi silver impregnation method,
courtesy of William W. Seeley, MD (*top*); Jerry and Cindy, courtesy of the
author (*bottom*).

All images are courtesy of the author unless otherwise noted.

*Special discounts are available for bulk purchases of this book. For more
information, please contact Special Sales at specialsales@jh.edu.*

Johns Hopkins University Press uses environmentally friendly book
materials, including recycled text paper that is composed of at least
30 percent post-consumer waste, whenever possible.

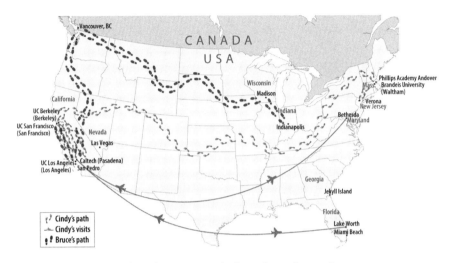

Cindy and Bruce's travels through North America.
Light gray footsteps are Cindy's. Dark gray footsteps are Bruce's.
Gray lines are Cindy's visits to her father, Jerry.

Drawing by Caroline Prioleau

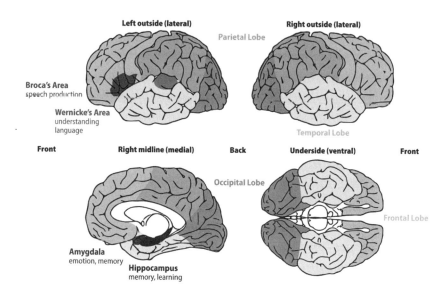

Key parts of the cerebral cortex.
Drawing by Caroline Prioleau

CONTENTS

A NOTE TO THE READER

You are about to read a sad story of a wonderful person, a father, whose cruel death by early-onset Alzheimer's disease took his daughter decades to recover from.* But you are also going to read a story, written with humor whenever possible, about finding solace through learning and sharing words. These words come from several worlds: neurology, literature, popular culture from the 1960s to the present, and a Jewish household where Yiddish was sprinkled in conversation like salt on brisket. We have tried to explain these terms as they arise in the chapters, but further definition seemed necessary, especially in the case of the medical vocabulary (and the Yiddish). Therefore, we have included a glossary at the end of the book. And although this book isn't meant to be a comprehensive discussion of dementia or a complete "how-to" guide for caregivers, we have also included images and tables that are meant to introduce readers to fundamental aspects of dementia, so that the first appointment with the neurologist (or general practitioner) isn't the first time they see these images or hear these words.

*Traditionally, a newly discovered disease is named in honor of the person recognized as the first person to describe it (for example, Alzheimer's disease). This practice leads to some ambiguity though (does the person have the disease or is the disease named for the person?). More modern usage tends to keep the name but drop the possessive form ("Alzheimer's disease" becomes "Alzheimer disease"). In this book, we have used the traditional possessive form, as this is how the diagnosis was delivered at the time.

Further explanation of literary references also seemed necessary. But unlike a neurological word that can be defined (a neuron, for example, is a nerve cell that transmits information), a book really can't be. Take *Moby-Dick*. Novel written by Herman Melville. 1851. One-legged captain tries to kill whale that bit off his leg. See what we mean? So, we have assembled the references to novels, poems, short stories, plays, neurological writings, etc. in a suggested readings section that follows the glossary. We hope that the literature mentioned, and the context provided in the chapters, makes you want to read (or reread) the books that have meant so much to us. Those works of the literary imagination, combined with the knowledge generated by the scientific imagination, have helped us find the right words. We hope they help you find yours.

I am fifty-eight years old, the age my father was when my mother called to tell me he had Alzheimer's disease. I am also in Berkeley, the same city I was in when I was twenty-five and got that phone call. A part of me has been frozen in that moment, even though over thirty years have intervened, during which time I got married, had two children, worked at Caltech (the California Institute of Technology), wrote some books, and went to my father's funeral.

I have returned to Berkeley to mourn the loss of my father—in Judaism, this is called sitting shiva—more than twenty years after he died. To say goodbye to him in the way I know best, which is to study, think, and write a book. I have always known that, unlike many memoirs about Alzheimer's disease, the book I would write about my father was one I wouldn't write alone. Having spent thirty years studying literature, I know that only someone who knows a field inside-out can explain its complexities in a way that can be understood by all readers. One year at the Memory and Aging Center (also known as the MAC) at the University of California, San Francisco (UCSF), learning about neurology would give me some familiarity with the science, but not nearly enough to write about it with the kind of expertise and clarity I believe is most helpful. Furthermore, I wanted a coauthor who could not only explain Alzheimer's disease but also share his knowledge with families dealing with other

kinds of neurological diseases, such as frontotemporal dementia (FTD) or Lewy body dementia. Last, the physicians who
accompanied my family through the years of my father's illness weren't much help. On the one hand, it was the 1980s, and
they didn't know much about the disease; on the other hand,
they had little interest in hearing how our family was manag-
ing. I wanted to write this book with a leading neurologist at
the cutting-edge of scientific research, so he could explain to
me what was happening to my father thirty years ago. That he
would listen and care so much was icing on the cake.

Thus, I asked Dr. Bruce Miller, founder of the MAC, to write
a book with me about dementia so I could tell the story of my
father's Alzheimer's disease, and he could explain the science
of dementia to people who may not have a degree in neurology. The argument of the book is implicit in its coauthorship:
that an interdisciplinary approach to Alzheimer's disease and
other dementias is the best way to help families dealing with
a life-changing diagnosis. Families are best cared for by sharing with them the emotional challenges as well as the scientific
ones. This is best done by integrating the perspectives of a family member and a physician. Through this process, the family
member gains knowledge about the neurology, thereby becoming more informed, confident in advocacy and caregiving,
and the doctor learns about the family's experiences, thereby
becoming more empathic, better able to understand their emotional needs.

What Bruce probably didn't know when he agreed to write
this book was that I was also asking him to sit shiva with me.
How could he, when I didn't know I was sitting shiva? But
his empathic embrace of my story and his willingness to use
it as a departure point to help others dealing with dementia
has allowed me to recover. To recover from some of the pain
of watching my beloved father become unglued and to recover

memories of him. Not lost on me is the irony of claiming that as my father lost memory, I did too.

The epigraph of my first book, written while my father was still alive, went like this: "For my mother and father, whose memory is safe in mine." Turns out, I could not keep Dad's memory safe, but I could keep my memories of him safe. In a strange twist of fate, though, I kept them safe by hiding them from myself. They were too precious, and I was too broken. I couldn't trust myself with them. Remembering the bad stuff was excruciating and remembering the good was even worse. Like fossils trapped in amber, they hardened and became stuck. I was stuck. This year, with Bruce, I found the strength to remember them. This book records those memories and tells the story of finding them.

In learning about how the brain works and how it becomes compromised, I was able to revisit what doctors call the clinical presentation—my father's words evaporating, for example— of my father's Alzheimer's disease. With this understanding and the passage of time, I could re-see those images of my father from a different vantage point, and, as my emphasis changed from my own sadness about my father's presentation to the presentation itself, I got clarity. A kaleidoscope provides a good analogy. It was as if Alzheimer's disease had broken my father into bits, and whenever I looked at my father through the kaleidoscope, I could only see the fragments he had become and how fragmented that made me feel. As the last part of that sentence suggests, for a very long time, I was only able to think about this disease from my own point of view. My loss of my father. My sadness. Studying neurology has been the adjustment to the kaleidoscope that I needed. Things have come into focus, with my father at the center of the story, where he belongs. This shift in perspective hasn't taken away the pain, as these chapters will make clear, but it has been profoundly beneficial. It has brought me closer to my father. I can remember him now.

By looking directly at the hardest memories, I have been able to find the happiest ones. And this is the structure of the book. It begins with the shock of the diagnosis, which Bruce responds to with a historical reflection on the changing nature of diagnosis, and the chapters work their way through the manifestations of the disease. Because my father's word-finding difficulties were his first symptom, that becomes the subject—an especially charged one for me because of my budding career as a literary scholar—for my exchange with Bruce about language and Alzheimer's. As my father's disease progressed, his sense of spatial orientation began to disintegrate, as did mine; that is, I lost track of my personal space, who I was. Bruce responds with a meditation on the profound effects on identity that happen with neurodegenerative disorders, both for the patient and their loved ones. Also, he describes why our spatial coordinates go awry with Alzheimer's disease. One of the last manifestations of my father's Alzheimer's had to do with his behavior, which included, to my mind, the most pronounced presentation of his depression: it took the form of a particular sound he made. One I hadn't remembered, or couldn't remember, because it was the sound of his suffering. Working through the memories of my father's Alzheimer's allows me to write the final chapter and get to the other side of his disease, to the time before he got sick. At last, I can remember him whole. In response, Bruce explains how memory works. Finally, I can tell those stories that I couldn't tell at that first shiva, in 1997.

The Jewish tradition of sitting shiva involves people coming to the house for several days, bringing lots of unhealthy but delicious food, and sharing memories of the person who died. When my father died at the age of seventy, having lost his memories, and much more, well before then, we sat shiva.

But it was all wrong. Telling happy stories about Dad before Alzheimer's disease struck seemed impossible, because our lives, his life, had become defined by his illness. Perhaps that is all the more reason to recall the good things. But collectively, we couldn't do it. The rabbi told an uninspiring allegory about dying and memory. I distinctly remember him taking a glass of water and pouring sugar into it, which then dissolved. We were the water. Dad was the sugar. Something like that, but I had already checked out, thinking that reading the beat poet Allen Ginsberg's "Kaddish," a poem about grieving for his dead mother, would have been more relevant. Maybe I should have listened to the rabbi more carefully. Or maybe I should have spent time with my children, Sarah and Sam, who at that time were three and one, and watched *The Lion King* on a continuous loop during those days Dad was dying and then while we were sitting shiva. I remember hearing the song "The Circle of Life" more than a few times and shrinking from the analogy between my experience and Simba's.

During those days of distorted mourning, my mother decided that she needed to sell the house that she and Dad had lived in. She couldn't bear staying in a place defined by pain and wanted to get out right away. And I mean right away. In between thanking people for bringing over platters of corned beef and cinnamon walnut *rugelach*, washing dishes, and pretending everything was okay, we were getting the house ready to put on the market. My mom would sell the house shortly after that and then move several times over in the course of the next several years. She couldn't find a place for herself. That she ended up with my family in California for her final years makes me extraordinarily happy. I couldn't, I didn't take care of my father, but I was able to take care of her. When she died, I held her in my arms. How I wish I had done that when my father was dying.

Usually, a family like mine sits shiva for a few days, attending

Friday night services to say kaddish, to say goodbye. Because I didn't get it right the first time, I needed a do-over. And because so many years have passed between his illness, his death, and my readiness to acknowledge what transpired over all of that time, I have needed to sit shiva for a year (which is actually what very religious Jews do). This is a long time, I know, but if you put something off for more than three decades, repairing the damages caused by delay can take a while. I'm like a flat tire that's been sitting in the shop waiting for the mechanic to fix it. I'm finally patched.

• •

Because I think in terms of literature, Herman Melville's Bartleby is the character who comes closest to capturing what my state of mind has been for all of these years. Published in 1853, "Bartleby, the Scrivener" tells the story of a worker whose job is to copy the legal documents his boss, the lawyer of the firm and the narrator of the story, asks him to. Initially, he is an ideal employee and then, out of the blue, starts refusing to do the work assigned to him by his boss.

In a sentence as famous as the opening of *Moby-Dick*'s "Call me Ishmael," Bartleby replies to his boss's requests with, "I would prefer not to." This preference, which is not an outright "no" but functions that way, drives the narrator to distraction. The story has some funny moments, such as when the narrator desperately suggests that Bartleby use his nonexistent conversational skills to become a traveling salesman, or when the narrator gets so frustrated with Bartleby's immobility (after having worked at a seemingly inhuman pace, Bartleby not only refuses to work but also refuses to leave the workplace) that the narrator moves into different law offices. The story also has some devastating moments. Bartleby becomes ghostlike as the story progresses. His body becomes an empty shell housing a lost soul who refuses all connection with the outside world until finally, the outside world takes him to prison for unlawfully occupying a space that is not his. At the end of the story, he dies facing a wall.

Like Bartleby, I had very strong preferences, the most important being that I would prefer not to see my father disappear before my very eyes. Therefore, I closed them, figuratively speaking. The other very important preference was that I wanted to read. Therefore, I opened them, literally speaking. Looking back, I see that a small part of my brain was open too, open to the possibility of getting glimpses of what was happening to my father without having to reckon with it directly. The two preferences came together in the following way: literature became a kind of crack—a window slightly open, a door slightly ajar—which my father's disease squeezed through. Sort of open and sort of closed. Simultaneously. That he would have preferred that I not give up my dream of reading and writing for a living did not make my decision to stick with it, all those years ago, any easier. I knew he wanted me to continue with my life, and not sacrifice it, even when he was directionless, speechless, and drugged-out in the nursing home.

But memories of my father—the catatonic one and the beautifully aware one—have been knocking at the door for a long while now, and I have known that I owe him a book. His love and selflessness made it possible for me to do what I love (read and write), and now I must return the gift. Obviously, I cannot give it to him, but I can give it to myself and anyone who chooses to read it. He would have wanted his experience to be recorded so that it could help others. Oddly, this has been the easy part: knowing that I had to write a book about him. It was a matter of finding the time and the right time.

With each academic book I have written, there has been this in-between time when I have thought, "Now I'll write the book about my dad." But for better or worse, I would have an idea about American literature that would prevent me (or I would allow myself to be prevented) from writing this more personal book.

My most recent monograph on American literature included the subtitle, *When Is Now?* Well, *now* is when I would no longer prefer to not look at my father's Alzheimer's. Let me put that awkward sentence, with its double negative, more positively: I would prefer to understand my father's dementia and my relation to it now. Why? Because now (at fifty-eight) is when I found out my father (at fifty-eight) was sick. Because now I can write this book about my father, for my father, with Bruce, who this year will be turning seventy, the same age as my father when he died. My memory is good; my grammar intact; my word-finding ability unimpaired. This may not always be the case.

• •

As anyone who has lost someone knows, the end of official grieving doesn't mean the end of grieving. That said, my year of sitting shiva—in Berkeley reading books, at UCSF studying neurology—has given me the chance to get it right. I can now remember my father without wanting to dissolve, and I have even retrieved some very happy and funny memories along the way. They are no longer fossilized. They have come alive in a series of chapters about diagnosis, language, spatial disorientation, behavior, and memory. While Bruce explains the neurology behind the clinical presentations I describe, he also reflects upon his career as a doctor and the values that have driven his commitment to understanding dementia and listening to families. This has helped me immensely, and I believe it will help others. Having remembered my father, having kept my word that he is safe in the pages of this book, I can at last say goodbye to him.

FINDING THE RIGHT WORDS

• I •

Diagnosis

Hitting the Fan

Early-onset Alzheimer's disease with the logopenic variant. That is
what my father had. It has taken me thirty years to get that
diagnosis, and this chapter will try to make sense of why it has
been so necessary for me to be able to write that sentence (well,
fragment—there is no verb), and how I have gone about finding those words and finding Bruce Miller, the person who gave
them to me.

This chapter will tell the story of how I have come to write
this book with Bruce about my father. The main arc begins with
me learning in 1985 that my father had been diagnosed with
Alzheimer's disease. It ends with me studying brain health in
2018 with Bruce and the many amazing neurologists, psychologists, neuropsychologists, psychiatrists, and caregivers at the
MAC at UCSF as an Atlantic Fellow at the Global Brain Health
Institute (GBHI). This book will fill in some of the blanks of
those thirty-three years, but will do so in a series of chapters
that are organized conceptually rather than in the temporal sequence that characterized my father's dementia. Thus, each
chapter starts with a particular moment in time—a memory,

sometimes more than one, that I have of my father losing an aspect of himself—and then zeroes in on it, using all my strength to remember how I understood those powerful and painful eruptions of my father's disease. I recall how literature gave me a way to look away from and look at (at the same time) what was happening to him. The memories are organized around my father's loss of language, his spatial confusion, and his behavioral changes. Chapter 5, "In Memoriam," describes the twenty-five years, give or take, I had with my healthy father before he developed Alzheimer's disease. Ironically, given the fact that my father had Alzheimer's disease, it was me, the cognitively healthy one, who had also forgotten those years. Only by going back to Berkeley, studying neurology, sitting shiva, and writing this book have I been able to recollect those precious details. Bruce's commentary follows each of my chapters. The nonsequential style of narration that I adopt is faithful to my memory of my father's memory, and as such doesn't lay out a precise timeline of my father's forgetting.

In this chapter, though, I will try to remember the order of his forgetting because chronology, or the putting together of a story into sequential order, plays an essential role in the diagnosis of dementia. I say "try" because my father was diagnosed with Alzheimer's disease in Lake Worth, Florida, while I was a graduate student in Berkeley, California. In other words, I was very far away and had a back-row seat to this horror show, but my memory of particular scenes is quite good. Bruce assures me that this sequence, even if it isn't exactly spot-on, needs to be told. An accurate diagnosis depends a lot on knowing what goes wrong when. What part of the brain gets hit first matters. For example, if the downward spiral begins with vision problems, the sick neuron probably lies somewhere in the occipital lobe, which may mean that the person has a visual variant of Alzheimer's disease known as Benson's syndrome. Things look blurry; objects within reach can't be grasped because the person can't see them.

In the language of literature, the order of events makes up the plot, which informs an interpretation; in the language of medicine, the order of the symptoms creates a plot of the disease, which in turn allows for a diagnosis. The best readers of stories help us see the importance of details in the plot that we may have overlooked or failed to appreciate. Literary critics use a strategy of "close reading" to unfold the complexities of a novel or a poem. Doctors do this, too, but what gets "closely read" are symptoms, such as shaky gaits, incomplete sentences, and wobbly handwriting. The brain also gets "read," as it were, in MRIs (magnetic resonance imaging) and PET (positron emission tomography) scans. These images of the brain don't reveal the symptoms but rather explain them with reference to the location of the atrophy, or shrinkage, in the brain. The best readers of MRIs can see where the sulci (grooves in the brain) are too deep or too wide, indicating erosion, or with the case of PET, the areas where metabolism is diminished. They can tell when the gyri (the folds in the brain) lose mass and get scrawny, signaling deterioration.

As an English professor and the daughter of a father who had early-onset Alzheimer's disease with the logopenic variant, I find this language of atrophy, aphasia, sulci, and logopenic variant at once powerful and weirdly comforting. I feel enriched by these words. Partly because learning new words—even ones that translate into pain—makes me happy. And partly because they tell a story about my father that, looking back, might have been valuable to me at the time he was ill. They exude accuracy and stability—so what if they are constructed and make sense only until the next discovery is made, and then they have to move over to make room for new words?—in contrast to the emotional quagmire of grief, love, and guilt with which I have been preoccupied for a very long time. It might have helped, even just a little bit, to have known that his losses had biological and chemical origins; that they weren't, or they weren't only, some sadistic act of a God that I didn't even believe in.

It never occurred to me to audit a neurology class at Berkeley and get some of these words then. Instead, I relied on what I knew (books, character, plot, identity) and what I was at Berkeley to know more about (American literature, nineteenth-century American culture, literary theory). This literary landscape provided an escape from and a container, bound between two covers, for an understanding of my father's suffering and my own. Exactly how this both worked and didn't will be explained in what follows. Suffice it to say that as a professional strategy, albeit an unconscious one, it was a winner. I got a good job doing what I loved. As a psychological strategy, not so great. A tremendous amount of mental energy, expended on a daily basis, went into shifting my attention from being devastated about my father to being focused on literature. Blocking entry by using literature as a "do not enter" sign worked wonders, as the only thing to fear were the words on the page, "The End." But all things must pass, as George Harrison said.

It's not, however, too late for me to learn and experience the value of another perspective—a scientific one—because even though my father died many years ago, grieving never ends. I suppose a cynical reader (do you see my hand going up?) might say that I am replacing one framework that kept my father's disease at a distance with another. Fair enough, but wrong. These new words are the building blocks of a conceptual apparatus that explains, but doesn't explain away, my father's symptoms. For example: he couldn't remember what he had for breakfast because his hippocampus was getting sick. Or, how grateful I am that he didn't have the behavioral variant of frontotemporal dementia because that would have meant that his capacity for empathy would have disappeared and his behavior would have been unrecognizable. Had he suffered from this kind of dementia, he might have laughed when my mother cried. He had early-onset Alzheimer's disease with the logopenic variant, but he was always my father. Loving, generous, present. The logopenic variant meant that he didn't have those words to tell me he loved me, that his love would never run out, that he would always be there (at least in my memory). But I always knew he knew me or remembered knowing me, and loved me or remembered loving me.

It's not that this medical/scientific framework would have replaced the one I had available (daughter/reader) in that summer of 1985, when I was just starting to study for my oral exams and was sitting at the kitchen table one evening in my studio apartment taking notes on Jonathan Edwards's 1741 Puritan sermon "Sinners in the Hands of an Angry God," when my mother called and told me that Dad had Alzheimer's disease; in fact, any semblance of a detailed, medical account of Alzheimer's wasn't available to doctors at that time. Besides, some of the things the doctors did say were pretty stupid. For example, when my father's hearing seemed to be giving him trouble, my mother took him to a hearing doctor sometime in the 1970s, the decade of feminists like Betty Friedan and Germaine Greer. After the testing had been completed, the doctor said that there was nothing wrong with my father's hearing. He then asked my mother how long they had been married and offered up this beauty of a piece of advice: "He just is tired of listening to you." Hearing difficulties can, of course, be related to cognitive ones. We also now know that the prodromal stage of dementia (when the disease is percolating, and certain symptoms may appear) can last for decades before a diagnosis.

So even if, in my twenties, it had occurred to me to ask my

father's neurologists about what was actually happening in his brain, they wouldn't have been able to say much. I do recall a doctor or two saying that there was no cure (that, sadly, remains the case), and a diagnosis of Alzheimer's disease with 100 percent certainty could only be made at an autopsy. This is no longer true because we have blood biomarkers as well as MRI and PET scans that illuminate the tau and amyloid proteins that asphyxiate the brain. Support for caregivers wasn't even mentioned, let alone discussed in a way that would have been informative or helpful. We were on our own; more precisely, my mother was on her own; and even more to the point, Dad was. Also, in the 1980s, all dementia was Alzheimer's disease, whereas now we know about a myriad of brain diseases, including frontotemporal dementia (a category that itself is multifaceted), dementia with Lewy bodies (what Robin Williams had), vascular dementia, and many others, with Alzheimer's disease being the most common. Learning this new language helps me understand my father better. This different approach to thinking about what makes a person a person gives me another lens through which to explain the time that began during that summer when I was twenty-five to that summer, thirteen years later, when he died. It brings me closer to him.

Exactly why I feel this way is difficult to pin down. The best I can do goes something like this: in getting inside of his brain, I can get outside of mine and get out of the way. I have been in the way for too long. To be honest, this other approach, thinking about what Alzheimer's disease does to the brain, for a moment takes my mind away from what is called the clinical presentation and how sad it made me feel. The science provides a kind of psychic reprieve. For example, I remember back to how my dad would whistle when he couldn't say a word— it would come out twisted. The whistle didn't have the well-defined musical sound and contour that Dad's whistles had in earlier times. This new, hoarse whistle lacked confidence and was often accompanied by a sad shake of the head and a look that asked for help. It acknowledged that he knew the word wasn't coming out right but offered the pretense that he had mispronounced it and could fix it the second time round. Remembering how the disease presented is still awful, of course, but early-onset Alzheimer's disease with the logopenic variant is about my father, specifically about the atrophy in his temporal-parietal lobes, which make up part of the incredibly complex circuitry of language production. This diagnosis is not about me watching his symptoms, taking note of their presentation, grieving, feeling bad about not dropping everything and moving back home to take care of him, understanding he wouldn't have wanted me to do that, and then back to square one. Rather this diagnosis is about him. But because I had no description of what was happening to him, I could only describe what was happening to me. And at a certain point, this self-description became a hall of mirrors, and I became stuck and needed more.

Perhaps if my career had been nurtured in a university with a religious sensibility, I would have explored religion as a way out (or way in) to a different and deeper understanding of my father's illness. Doubt it. But because for the last thirty years or so I have breathed in an atmosphere that produced the Mars Rover and Planet 9, several Nobel laureates, and lord knows how many patents, science beckoned and seemed the logical door of perception that I needed to go through. I can imagine the puzzlement of my Caltech colleagues when I offer the following reflection: what I value about the science of the brain, among many things, is that it is about my father. In a fundamental way that I suspect may sound strange, studying the brain is, for me, studying my father's brain. Granted, the four lobes that define the cerebral cortex do not capture the whole picture. The brain is more than the temporal, parietal, frontal, and occipital lobes; my father was more than his brain, but if you're going to pick one organ, that seems like an excellent one to choose. And that's where this other way of understanding my father and his illness comes into play.

Now I get to do both. This book brings together both, and by both, I mean many things. The both of 1985 and 2018; the both of me and Bruce; the both of literature and neurology; the both of my healthy father and my sick father. Studying the workings of the brain brings my father back to me so I can go over (knowing there is no do-over) those years, especially when he was sick, and get a better idea of what was going on—not with me, but with him. And the best part of it all is I don't have to be alone. I can do this with a doctor I trust, one who will stay with me and explain why my father lost his words; why my father pointed his three-iron golf club toward the swimming pool and not the putting green; why he couldn't recognize my mother. I get to ask and ask again (one of the mantras of science is that there are no stupid questions) all of those questions that I was too traumatized to ask in my twenties, but which the doctors couldn't have answered anyway, and get some answers. I can revisit those years. Not as a frightened daughter and graduate student committed to getting a job as an English professor, come hell or high water (who knew there would be so much hell?), but rather as a still somewhat frightened adult (plus a husband, two kids, minus both parents) and feisty academic determined to understand some modicum of biology and chemistry. I want to share this story in order to help others—family members, caregivers, people experiencing mild cognitive impairment—dealing with the emotional pain of Alzheimer's disease.

But I cannot tell this story of my father by myself, nor do I want to. One's memoir, as any editor will tell you, does not usually require two authors. Why does this one have to/two? The first reason has to do with the science and my background as an academic. Bruce, who majored in English and education as an undergraduate at the University of Madison, Wisconsin, has spent a career becoming one of the most prominent researchers in brain health. He is a beautiful close reader, who has studied the paintings made by his patients with frontotemporal dementia and tracked the development of the disease in relation to changes in the color, outline, and form of their artworks. He links Emily Dickinson's ability to represent mental states to neurologists' ideas about the brain. He loves to write.

Bruce and I met in his office at the MAC during the summer of 2017 on the recommendation of Kenneth Kosik, a neurologist at the University of California, Santa Barbara, who also majored in English and received a master's degree in it before deciding to go into neurology. I found Ken through David Baltimore, one of those Nobelists to whom I was referring earlier. The conversation with Bruce quickly turned to our favorite works of literature. Although Bruce loves Thomas Pynchon (Ken does, too; in fact, his master's thesis was on Pynchon), and I don't, this didn't seem fatal. Just a difference in taste. That said, I confess to being somewhat taken aback when, after our first meeting, in which Bruce recommended that I read Pynchon's *Inherent Vice*, and I then went home and dutifully read it, I wondered why a book on sex, drugs, and rock 'n' roll was a favorite of his, and what this might say about him, what he thought it might say about me, and what it might mean for our coauthorship. Turns out, it meant very little other than that we're both hippies at heart. I, of course, suggested he take another look at *Moby-Dick*.

In Bruce, I have found someone who studies empathy and the brain. Someone who is so empathic that even though he only knows my father through my writing, agreed to take on my father's case (and mine), even though my father is dead. And there are no MRIs. In that initial conversation, Bruce asked me whether we had any images of my father's brain, and I had to break the news that no, we didn't. I had called the neurologist's office in Bethesda, Maryland, whose name and address I instantly recognized when I googled "neurology Bethesda." I remember that office on Wisconsin Avenue and having an awful family meeting (sometime in the late 1980s) in it. I do not remember what was specifically said all those years ago, but in 2018, when I spoke to the nurse, she said the records were so old that they no longer had them. Bruce said it didn't matter. He knew what my father had, to which I replied, "How?" He said, "By the age of your father's onset, by what you've written, and by your reaction to your father when you talk about him." I guess people who have loved ones with early-onset Alzheimer's disease exude a particular kind of grief, which Bruce, in his decades-long work on brain health, has seen many times before. I haven't cried in front of Bruce but was pretty close at that moment.

But back to the science and why I have asked Bruce to write this book with me. Just as I have spent years studying literature, Bruce brings years of scientific expertise to this project, and because of that, he can talk about the science in a way that only an expert, who understands the material inside-out, can to a general audience. It was crucial for me to find someone who could do with the science what I wanted to do with the literature. If we have written this right, the reader needn't be an English professor or a neurologist to find something of value in these chapters. Just someone trying to make sense out of the experience of living with a loved one who has a neurological disease.

That explains why I can't write this book alone. Why I don't want to is a more complicated matter. Part of the answer lies in the loneliness of writing and not wanting to be alone when I write this particular book. When I am alone and happily writing about Edgar Allan Poe, for example, who teases the reader with a narrator who seems reliable but is out of his mind, I do not find myself crying. However, I cry when I write about the recollection of my father no longer knowing how to load the film in the camera (once upon a time, when a person had to do that). Writing with Bruce helps. Putting my father, and my memories of him, in Bruce's hands, feels safe. Another and related answer has to do with the loneliness of grieving. At twenty-five, I was consumed with grief but didn't share it—even with myself. I was too busy protecting myself and others from its power, which I was certain would destroy everything in its wake. Thirty-some-odd years later, the obvious fact that some things are just too hard to do alone has finally gotten through. I don't have to write this story of my father's dementia by myself. I already lived it by myself (not literally, of course, but it often felt that way), and so, why do that again? I needed someone then, and I need someone now. And last, I don't want to write this book alone because it will be better for having Bruce's voice in it. What I mean by better is richer, smarter, wiser. I would have been richer, smarter, and wiser had I the benefit of Bruce's voice many years ago, so why not hear it now and share it with others who don't have the good fortune to study neurology with him? Solos are fine, but duets can be finer.

• •

Not lost on me is the fact that I am failing to provide the chronology that I initially promised so that Bruce can write about the process of diagnosis. Let me try again.

The scene is the summer of 1982. Dad and I have flown together from our home state of New Jersey to California. We land at LAX and spend the night at the home of cousins who live in Encino. There had been a fabulous deal at an L.A.

Toyota dealership, and my cousin picked up the rust-colored, two-door stick shift Tercel that my parents had bought for me. The plan was for me and Dad to take our time and drive up the Pacific Coast Highway, also known as the PCH or the 1 (California freeways, like people, have nicknames), the scenic freeway that runs along the Pacific Ocean from Orange County to the Bay Area.

I was driving, which now strikes me as odd, but at the time didn't. Dad told me smilingly that it was my car, so I should drive. With the benefit of hindsight, I wonder, was he covering up something? Did he not want to drive? Had the prodromal stage of the disease, those years when the neurons begin to go rogue, but the brain can still carry on, already begun? We stayed on the 1 for an hour or two, at which point, Dad got scared. He wanted to go inland where the terrain was flat. I suggested that maybe he would be happier if he drove. After all, he loved to drive, and back in the day, as in only a year before, he had thought nothing of picking me up at the end of one of my undergraduate semesters at Brandeis University by noon (the ride from Verona, New Jersey to Waltham, Massachusetts was about five hours) and returning home by 6 p.m., in time for dinner. If Dad were having flashbacks to teaching me how to drive a stick shift, I couldn't blame him for being concerned. The grinding, the stalling, the rolling back and forth at the top of hills. It wasn't pretty. That my clutch skills had improved significantly was beside the point.

So, when I asked him if he wanted to drive, I thought for sure he would say yes, and that would solve his worry that I was going to take a hairpin turn too fast and drive us off a cliff. But no, he wanted to scrap our itinerary, which included staying in a kitschy room at the famous Madonna Inn in San Luis Obispo, and get away from those winding roads and their danger signs. The height of the freeway compared to the drop to the ocean did give me a lump in my throat, but unlike Dad, I was reluctant to concede defeat. We argued about it a little (he was such a good driver, why wouldn't he want to take the wheel?), but then pointed the car toward Bakersfield. Looking back, I think maybe this was the first sign of something wrong. I don't remember Dad being afraid of anything, especially when it came to driving. And I don't remember him not following through on a plan, especially one that he had been excited about.

The danger signs on the PCH were clearly both literal and figurative. Dad and I, but really Dad, were in danger of something far worse than either of us could have imagined. There were other warning signs that I should have seen, that I wish I had seen, during that trip to California when Dad dropped me off at Berkeley. All I could see and feel, though, was the promise of freedom that coursed through my body that first time we were on the 80 freeway and the University Avenue exit for Berkeley came into view.

Before I get to the moment when we said goodbye at the San Francisco Airport where Dad cried, and I chalked it up to him missing me and not him starting to miss himself, let me share some funny anecdotes about my father, me, and Berkeley. It's the spring of 1982 and I get accepted into the PhD program. We are sitting on a bench in Verona Park, and Dad reads the acceptance letter. He's proud; however, that letter of congratulations includes another page with a graph of the number of people who applied for jobs in English over a ten-year period (or was it five?) and the percentage who got jobs. The numbers were dreadful, and Dad turned to me and said, "Why don't you go to law school like your sister and brother?" I explained why (the reasons will become clear in the chapters that follow), he shook his head, and when the time came for me to go to California, he was all in. Buying me a car said as much.

But when push came to shove, it was hard for him to let go, even though he bought me the wheels that gave me the license to leave. Speaking of licenses, I have a funny story about going to the Oakland DMV with Dad in order to get my California driver's license. Having driven for several years prior to my arrival in Berkeley, I was uncharacteristically cocky. I tend to overstudy for tests, but not this time. I didn't take even a few minutes to review the dingy-gray, twenty-five-page-or-so driver's manual on the wall at the DMV. Big mistake, because I could not remember the right number of car lengths you were supposed to maintain behind the car in front of you (as if people paid any attention to that on the California freeways) or how to make a right turn so as not to run over the bicyclist in the bicycle lane to your right, or when to use the fog lights versus the bright lights versus the dim lights. To my astonishment, I failed the written test. Dad was incredulous, too. I barely passed the second time. Making one more mistake would have meant another failure.

And speaking of failures, here's another funny story. I tell it because the climax is about messing up letters and getting the words wrong and getting a taste, though I didn't know it at the time, of my father's relentless battle with vowels and consonants. The scene is the *Wheel of Fortune* stage in Burbank, California in, I think it was, 1986. There had been a call for college students to try out for a spot on the show, and the talent scouts came to Berkeley. I had been an avid and successful *Wheel of Fortune* player from the safety of various dens with televisions in New Jersey, Florida, and California, and so decided to try out for the show, even though I was a graduate student. Trained from an early age in the arts of Scrabble, Boggle, and hangman, I could often solve the puzzles with little more than one or two letters showing on the big board. I was one of three students selected to represent UC Berkeley and was soon on the way to L.A. to compete. On the day of taping, each student had to wear their school's sweatshirt. Mine was a light gray with the Berkeley letters in white. My parents flew out from Florida to watch and cheer me on. My Berkeley friends came to my apartment for a send-off party, where we took turns talking about what Vanna would wear and Shakespeare.

I was nervous as hell by the time game day came around, more so than when I took my oral exams, a difficult rite of passage (more on this in another chapter) en route to getting a PhD. The whole vibe of the thing threw me off. First, if we had to use the bathroom, someone from the show had to accompany us lest we cheat. I wasn't used to being treated with such suspicion. Second, the makeup people put heavy pancake powder on my face and that made me uncomfortable. I don't wear makeup, and when I asked one of the makeup people if it might be possible to dispense with the foundation that felt like I had another face on top of my real face, she told me no. Last, Pat looked scary with all of his makeup that turned his face into a mask, plus his attitude toward us players seemed robotic. Apparently, I was so nervous that in the tape recording of the show, which was made by my boyfriend Jim's parents, who were later to become my in-laws, I was holding my hands on the podium rocking back and forth not unlike the back and forth motion of the people in temple silently saying their prayers. These movements are called davening. Jim found this disconcerting and, in an act of great generosity that I am not sure I would have been able to pull off had the positions been reversed, never insisted that I watch it with him. I did watch the tape once, alone, years later. Thankfully, DVD players and Blu-rays have replaced video recorders, and so the evidence of my shame can't be easily retrieved. Plus, I made sure the VHS

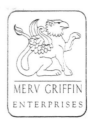

Dear Cindy:

Congratulations on being chosen to represent your
school during WHEEL OF FORTUNE's College Week.

Please contact the following team members in order
to prepare a 30-45 second talk about your school.
If your team makes the final cash round, one person
will be selected to represent the team. As no one
knows who that will be, everyone must learn the same
information:

Stephanie Burke   548-6206
Lyn Christopulos   644-2725
Douglas Young   849-4492

College Week will be taped on Saturday May 3, 1986
One person will come back on Sunday May 4, 1986
to participate on a syndicated show.

See you soon.

Sincerely,
WHEEL OF FORTUNE

Harv Selsby
Contestant Coordinator

HS/nle

— Please Reply To: —

| MERV GRIFFIN PRODUCTIONS EXECUTIVE OFFICES 1541 N. Vine St. Hollywood, CA 90028 (213) 461-4701 | TRANS-AMERICAN VIDEO, INC. 1541 N. Vine St. Hollywood, CA 90028 (213) 466-2141 | TAV/COMMAND VIDEO, INC. 1541 N. Vine St. Hollywood, CA 90028 (213) 466-2141 | TAV/SOUND, INC. 6200 W. 3rd. St. Los Angeles, CA 90036 (213) 937-2460 |

Divisions of Merv Griffin Enterprises

Congratulatory letter to Cindy, informing her of her upcoming participation
in *Wheel of Fortune*'s 1986 "College Week"

cassette stayed on top of the dryer in the laundry room for
many, many years, accumulating dust, absorbing heat, and
gradually self-destructing (well, destructing with my help).

It was my turn to spin the wheel, which had looked easy
on Channel 4 but was hard in person. The real experience of

playing the game was already different, and not in a good way, from watching the show on TV. Vanna had turned over some letters—maybe the S and the N—that had been called by the first player, who then hit the bankrupt slot on the wheel. The puzzle had a lot more letters in it, and I had plenty of time to make some money. In a flash, I knew the answer and could taste victory. The trip to Puerto Vallarta, which would have been one of the prizes had I won, was in my grasp. Only one question remained: should I take my mom who desperately needed a vacation from my dad, or Jim with whom I wanted to go to Mexico?

To capture the complete humiliation of this moment, it is necessary to introduce a seemingly unrelated fact. Jim, a graduate student in the classics department, who, like me, would go on to get his PhD, and for some inexplicable reason loved the television show *Miami Vice*. Another NBC success story. The chapters that follow will reveal my ambivalence about the state of Florida—the location of my grandma Sarah's death and my father's—which irrationally extended to that particular show. By contrast is *Dexter*, a show I liked a lot because of its resonances with Poe. Also, *Dexter* had a realism that *Miami Vice* lacked, by which I mean that *Dexter* captured some of the more problematic aspects of Florida that I had identified: its humidity, where one's glasses instantly fog up when they encounter the oppressiveness of the outside air, and its menacing landscape, where children who played too close to the swampy waters that divide one condominium complex from another get eaten up by alligators lying in wait. In particular, I responded to *Dexter*'s linkage of serial killing and Florida. Thus, when Jim would watch *Miami Vice*, I would make fun of him for it. The whole show seemed stupid and poorly written (did anyone ever sweat?), and I found the names of the main characters, played by Don Johnson and Philip Michael Thomas, especially absurd: Sonny Crockett and Ricardo Tubbs. I would jeer at those names.

Do you know those people who say, "Pat, I would like to solve the puzzle," and then do so only to get one letter wrong and the audience kind of gasps or moans in disbelief, combined— at least in my case—with an air of superiority? I had always made fun of the contestants who attempted and failed to solve the puzzle, putting them down from my comfortable position on the sofa. Kind of like watching an ice-skater fall on her tush. Now I was one of them. I picked the T and, because there were three, added quite a bit to my stash. Not wanting to be greedy or hit the bankrupt sign, I went in for the kill and said the magic words I had heard hundreds of others say before: "Pat, I would like to solve the puzzle." He told me to go ahead, and I gleefully blurted out, "Sonny Crocker and Ricardo Tubbs." A ripple of something not quite right—like the smell of a fart when it first begins to reach consciousness—entered the atmosphere sur- rounding me, and Pat said, "I'm afraid that's not right," and went to the next contestant.

I couldn't watch *Wheel of Fortune* for years after that because of flashbacks (I remember wishing that I had passed out and the ambulance had come and the whole experience would dis- appear) and the karmic appropriateness of my verbal mistake. All those years I had made fun of those losers. All those years I had laughed at Pat Sajak's name. I found it humorous that his last name contained the word "say"—the "sa" pronounced as "say"—so on the occasions when *Wheel of Fortune* came up in conversation and Pat's name was mentioned, I would say, "Pat say jack jack." I was being punished for all those times I had told Jim what a dumb show *Miami Vice* was and laughed at the protagonists' names. My parents felt bad for me, and I for them, for shlepping out to California to see me fail, but by this point, unlike the DMV debacle, Dad didn't fully register my abjection. My mistake, saying R instead of T, was born of arrogance. How could I have mangled the words? I loved words and the letters out of which they were made. My father's difficulties with consonants were an altogether different matter. He didn't have a condescending bone in his body.

• •

Yet again, the story of my father's diagnosis has gone off the chronological rails. Let me try again and go back to that summer of 1982 when I was twenty-one and he was forty-six. If fear, sadness, and anxiety qualify as initial symptoms leading to a diagnosis of early-onset Alzheimer's with the logopenic variant, my chronology of Dad's illness begins in 1982, three years before the diagnosis. My guess is my mother's version would start with that hearing test years before. Who knows?

During those three years from 1982 to 1985, other symptoms accumulated before my mother told me Dad had Alzheimer's disease. It's worth pointing out that I don't really know when she got the diagnosis. I got it in 1985, which is why I began this chapter saying that its arc begins in that year. I remember asking her on the telephone that night exactly when she found out that Dad had Alzheimer's, and instead of replying to the direct question, she responded, "I was hoping not to tell you the diagnosis until you finished your degree." Like so many other things, I wish I had followed up. When did Mom know? I was too busy being angry about information withheld to press further. Of course, she was trying to protect me (as she always had) from the diagnosis, and, looking back, she had good reason to worry about me getting through Berkeley knowing that Dad had Alzheimer's disease. She wanted me to do what I loved. She, too, was very proud of my getting into Berkeley and maybe even proudest of all. Although she didn't go to college, she loved words and shared that love with me. But the idea that Dad would have Alzheimer's, and I wouldn't or shouldn't know it until such time as I completed my dissertation, is/was patently absurd. That I wouldn't figure out—from the monosyllabic replies on the telephone to the broken handwriting to the sight of the bedroom in Florida that looked like a war zone because Dad could no longer sleep—that something was terribly wrong seems crazy. But we all went crazy when Dad lost his mind, so I guess there's a logic to it.

Dad and I didn't get along those few days in California, which was weird. Conflict arose around where to go for dinner and the hotel we stayed in. But the moment that haunts me most is our goodbye at the airport. Dad cried and held me tight and trembled. I don't think I cried. I was happy to be in Berkeley and besides, we would be seeing each other over winter break, and I told him that it was only a few months away. That didn't help. Why was I always problem-solving instead of taking in the problem? I got to thinking that maybe this was less about a winter break and more about a bigger break. I tried to calm down Dad (why?) by reminding him of my promise that I would return to the East Coast after finishing my degree (an assurance that was stupid to make because of that graph about the job market, but nevertheless one that I could have kept, but didn't). He still cried. Why didn't I ask him why he was crying? Another opportunity to get close, and I whiffed.

At the time, I remember not really understanding why he cried. I am devastated by his tears and the fact that I didn't ask him to tell me why he seemed so inconsolable, especially now that I have done what was asked of me and put his symptoms into chronological order and must confront the fact (the interpretation?) that everything I needed to know was right in front of me in 1982 at the airport. But I was too blind, young, selfish, and happy to see it. As a result, I understood or misunderstood that goodbye and chalked up his sadness to him missing me because I'd be far away. Nothing more, nothing less.

Now, I know or think I know that the separation he dreaded had begun, and he knew it. Our goodbye wasn't about me at all. It was about him. For all of my talk about returning to him, he would not be able to return to me. We had gone inland, but he was already falling off the cliff. My turn would come a few years later.

The Detective Story

Considering the time, it is not surprising that Cindy's father never received a comprehensive assessment. In 1983, standard of care for the evaluation of cognitive symptoms was a brief visit with a physician, two to five minutes for the history and assessment, followed by a cold goodbye and good luck. We now know that difficulties with participating in and following conversations can, though of course not always, presage cognitive difficulties. It's not that the person can't hear; rather, they can't comprehend what they're hearing. Jerry heard but didn't fully understand. Most likely, the prodromal stage had begun. While diagnosis has improved substantially since 1983, in most settings, even now, dementia screening rarely happens, dementia assessments are cursory, and little support is offered to the patient or to their family once a diagnosis is made.

Diagnosis well, that has been my passion, my *raison d'être*, and ultimately, my unique (albeit small) contribution to the field of dementia. In medical school, at the University of British Columbia, I considered a career in many different medical specialties, including rural medicine, neurosurgery, cardiology, oncology, and infectious diseases. I loved them all, and my uncertainty about the right career path led me to take two years of internal medicine training after my graduation. During that time, I decided that neurology, with its detective-style history taking, its precise examination, and its relentless focus on diagnosis, was what I wanted to do for the rest of my life. Subspecialty training in behavioral neurology became a certainty, and in 1981, I left Canada and came to the University of California, Los Angeles, with the hope of working with the famous behavioral neurologist Frank Benson.

Behavioral neurology studies the drivers of our behavior, the intricate organization of language and speech, the anatomical basis for memory, navigation, executive function, moral reasoning, empathy, personality, and the self, as well as the evolution of behavior. This subspecialty touches on who we are, where we came from as a species, and why we do what we do. In retrospect, I would have gone almost anywhere to work with Frank. I might even have worked for free if he had asked me to. When I finished neurology training in 1983, my dream came true when Frank accepted me into the UCLA behavioral neurology fellowship. Remarkably, I did get paid, learned behavioral neurology in an incredible environment, and was introduced to a world of intellectuals with a passion for understanding how the brain worked and to find therapies for neurodegenerative disorders. Opportunity, foresight, fate, dumb luck, or whatever force or spirit led me to UCLA was beneficent and wise.

It has been more than twenty years since Frank's premature death from prostate cancer in 1996, and I still think about him nearly every day. Frank was a remarkable man who made it possible for me to succeed in the tough world of neurology. He taught me an approach to dementia that was smart and many years ahead of its time. Equally important, I learned to pursue openness to new people and ideas, restraint around the expression of one's convictions, and kindness to colleagues and patients, qualities that were not universally admired when I was training.

Frank's path to behavioral neurology reflected his confidence and passion. Working as a neurologist in a successful Oregon private practice, in 1965 Frank packed up his family and moved to Boston in order to start over as a fellow and to train with the father of behavioral neurology, Norman Geschwind. Frank became Geschwind's colleague, friend, and collaborator, and he quickly developed a reputation as a superb clinician and a solid but idiosyncratic researcher. Outstanding clinician, there was no doubt, and Frank might have been the premier clinician of his generation, successfully integrating his training in family practice and his knowledge of anatomy and neurology. He had a unique perspective on the psychiatric manifestations of neurological conditions. Enthusiasm for his research in academic neurology was more muted, as he tended to frame his ideas about brain-behavior relationships on single cases, an approach that was unpopular then, and still is today. Further, Frank never wrote grant proposals, believing that the review system was myopic and stifling to his creativity. Frank said about himself that he was a searcher, not a researcher. I think he meant that he wanted to discover new things and not get trapped in boring methodology.

Yes, his research was unconventional, but in Frank's defense, his powers of observation were keen, and he was rarely wrong. From single cases, Frank made bold and sweeping conclusions about brain organization that were often groundbreaking and important and still remain cogent more than fifty years later. This happened without a single dollar of funding from the National Institutes of Health.

Always a Westerner at heart and never totally at home on the East Coast, in 1979 Frank moved to UCLA to establish a behavioral neurology program. When I arrived as a resident in Los Angeles in 1981, Frank had just recruited his protégé Jeffrey Cummings to join him at UCLA. Jeff was recently out of his residency in Boston, where he had trained with Frank. Jeff, like Frank, was an extraordinary clinician and dementia theoretician. Only expecting Frank when I came to UCLA, I got Jeff as well. Jeff and Frank's book *Dementia: A Clinical Approach*, published in that same year, was the first comprehensive effort to clinically and pathologically delineate the different types of dementia, and it codified an approach to diagnosis that changed medicine. Not all dementia is caused by Alzheimer's disease, but Alzheimer's is a cause of dementia; in other words, "dementia" is the broad neurological term for the collection of symptoms caused

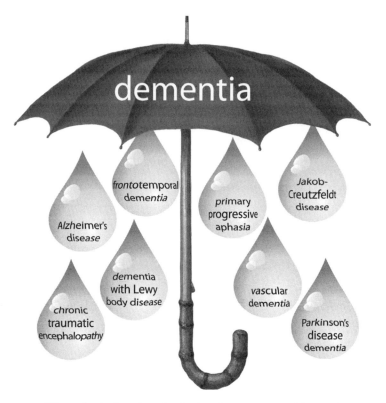

Different brain disorders that lead to the symptoms of dementia.
Drawing by Caroline Prioleau

by various brain diseases. Sadly, this more accurate and nuanced approach never touched Jerry Weinstein.

Frank was originally from North Dakota, and Jeff from Wyoming, and they were a refreshing contrast to the tough, elitist, East Coast figures who dominated neurology during the 1970s, '80s, and '90s. When I met Frank and Jeff, most academics believed that neurology was meant to deal with stroke, seizures, brain tumors, or peripheral nerve and muscle disorders, and they scorned cognitive neurology and dementia assessment. Egalitarian and charismatic, Frank and Jeff were buoyantly friendly and zealous populists in a world where elitism, contempt, and emotional restraint reigned. The two became highly effective advocates for both neurology and behavioral neurology, gathering devotees across the world!

A tall Clint Eastwood look-alike, Frank was brilliant, quick witted, and profoundly confident, yet his self-effacing sense of humor and gentle demeanor made him an approachable and universally respected leader. Jeff, tall and thin, with long hair and a black goatee, was serious, measured, soft-spoken, and formal. At first glance, Jeff seemed austere, and he looked like a cross between the American Old West frontiersman Wild Bill Hickok and Abraham Lincoln, but his blue-striped suits made it clear that he respected academic medicine. Jeff was open and gentle with a distinct and disarming laugh. Over time his hair got shorter, the suits and ties became more elegant. Eventually, he abandoned his beard. Diligent, relentlessly intellectual, and truly creative, Jeff had a passion for understanding the brain and teaching others what he learned. He was the first behavioral neurologist to exclusively focus on the dementias, and he opened himself to anyone with a similar interest. Jeff could draw the brain on command, often using both hands together, simultaneously sketching the brain stem and cerebellar hemispheres with the overlying cortical mantle. Like Frank, Jeff quickly became revered, particularly in Europe and Asia. Years later, my Greek neurologist friend John commented that watching Jeff speak at a meeting was like watching the Pope descend into a crowd where masses of people clamored to kiss his ring.

It was an exhilarating time to train at UCLA. In addition to their individual brilliance, Frank and Jeff attracted around them a creative collection of linguists, anthropologists, psychologists, and basic scientists, creating an electric and ever-evolving environment at the UCLA program. My peers, the other UCLA fellows, Michael Mahler, Stephen Read, Artiss Powell, Kyle Boone, Mario Mendez, and I, all became academics, and we knew that we were learning something that had never been taught before. In addition, Frank and Jeff imbued us all with skills and self-confidence that have lasted throughout our careers. They revealed the mysteries of the brain and translated them in a practical manner that was highly relevant to our patients. Important for me, Jeff and Frank encouraged me to study frontotemporal dementia, which became my lifetime passion. With the help of Jeff and Frank at UCLA and a unique group of young investigators at UCSF, where I moved to in 1998, it became possible to advance the understanding of FTD, at the time a mysterious, largely overlooked neurodegenerative condition, which is now at the forefront of diagnosis and therapy in the dementia field.

During that time, neurologists, psychiatrists, and internists were just beginning to discover that dementia was important, but still, in most settings, anyone who suffered from progressive cognitive impairment was diagnosed with Alzheimer's disease. By contrast, Frank and Jeff had a unique approach, devoted to the fidelity of clinical diagnosis and tracking that diagnosis back to the pathology in the brain. Calling all dementia Alzheimer's disease simplified (essentially eliminated) the diagnostic process and set the field back by ignoring the treatable causes for dementia, like vitamin deficiency, infection, metabolic disorders, medication reactions, etc. Frank and Jeff called these the reversible dementias. Also, by lumping non-Alzheimer's dementias, such as frontotemporal dementia and dementia with Lewy bodies, into the Alzheimer's basket, the rich variability of presentation and cause for cognitive impairment was missed. The death-knell for the "all dementia is Alzheimer's disease approach" came only recently, when billion-dollar clinical trials designed to lower the amyloid protein associated with Alzheimer's disease discovered that many patients, up to 36 percent in some trials, did not have amyloid in the brain, part of the standard pathological definition of Alzheimer's disease. They had been misdiagnosed, severely tainting the likelihood that the trials would have been successful, even if the compounds truly worked!

The history of dementia research has been a tale of progress,

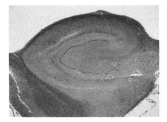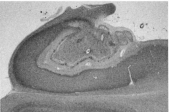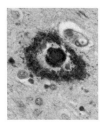

Normal hippocampus (*left*); hippocampus with neurofibrillary tangles staining dark (*center*); amyloid plaque (*right*). Plaques and tangles are the pathological hallmark of Alzheimer's disease.
Courtesy of Salvatore Spina, MD, PhD, of the
UCSF Neurodegenerative Disease Bank

quiescence and backsliding, and then progress again. The major neurodegenerative diseases were characterized clinically and pathologically at the turn of the twentieth century. Described by Alois Alzheimer in 1906, Alzheimer's disease is a progressive cognitive disorder with prominent memory loss associated with amyloid plaques and neurofibrillary tangles. Papers by Nicole Berchtold and Carl Cotman, as well as Michel Goedert have clarified that Czech neuropsychiatrist Oskar Fischer was as important as Alois Alzheimer in the description of the disease now almost exclusively associated with Alzheimer. History can be cruel and unfair with recognition for contributions sometimes tainted by power, friendships, political status, and even bigotry, influencing who gets proper credit and who does not. With the advent of the Oskar Fischer Prize and other efforts, Fischer is being elevated again to the status that he deserves.

Arnold Pick reported on patients with progressive language or behavioral disorders associated with frontotemporal atrophy in 1892, and this disorder is now called frontotemporal dementia. In 1910, a colleague of Alzheimer, Fritz Heinrich Lewy, described concentric neuronal inclusions that stain pink with an H&E stain, a finding characteristic of Parkinson's disease. This flurry of seminal discoveries about the clinical and pathological features of non-Alzheimer's dementias was followed by a dark ages that lasted nearly sixty years when little new was added to our knowledge about dementia, when the precision-medicine approaches of Alzheimer, Pick, and Lewy were forgotten, and dementia became synonymous with senility and arteriosclerosis, or vascular injury to the brain.

Renewed interest in dementia occurred during the 1970s, when British scientists Gary Blessed, Bernard Tomlinson, and Martin Roth reported that the severity of cognitive impairment of patients in nursing homes strongly correlated with the brain's concentration of amyloid plaques and neurofibrillary tangles. Suddenly, a dementing condition rarely seen in people under the age of sixty, Alzheimer's disease became the major cause for cognitive impairment in older adults. In 1975, Robert Katzman, a neurologist at Albert Einstein University, incorporated this information into a profoundly influential paper in which he reported upon an epidemic of dementia that was caused by what he called Alzheimer's disease, and the concept of senility had disappeared. Dementia and Alzheimer's disease were featured in *Time* magazine, and the concept that all dementia was Alzheimer's, flawed as this concept proved to be, became democratized.

In the 1980s and '90s, the different pathological lesions described by Alzheimer, Pick, and Lewy were precisely sequenced. The amyloid plaque in Alzheimer's disease consisted of a 42-amino-acid protein called amyloid-beta-42, while the neurofibrillary tangle was made up of twisted fibrils of a protein called tau. Abnormal clumps of protein found included within the cells of patients with frontotemporal dementia consist of one of two main proteins, either the Pick body (made of tau) or Pick-like inclusions (made of TDP-43). Another type of "inclusion," the Lewy body, was sequenced in 1997 and consists of a protein alpha-synuclein. Alzheimer's disease, frontotemporal dementia, and the parkinsonian dementias are the three main disorders that afflict our elderly population, with many patients seen in

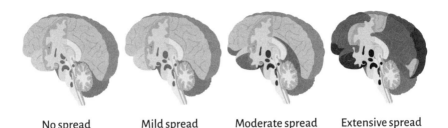

No spread   Mild spread   Moderate spread   Extensive spread

The spread of the misfolded form of the protein tau along functional networks
due to Alzheimer's disease.
Illustration courtesy of Cathrine Petersen

dementia clinics suffering from one of these conditions. That is the challenge of differential diagnosis, determining which one of these conditions is afflicting our patients. These discoveries set the stage for better diagnosis and ultimately treatment for dementia.

Amyloid-beta-42, tau, and alpha-synuclein, the proteins that aggregate in Alzheimer's disease, frontotemporal dementia, and Parkinson's disease, misfold and then spread across the brain by moving from one neuron to the next, killing the neurons that they have touched.

The discovery of protein misfolding and spread in dementia was made by UCSF neurologist Stanley Prusiner, and for these findings he received the Nobel Prize for Medicine in 1997. In Alzheimer's disease, the tau protein spreads from the hippocampus into the posterior temporal-parietal cortex, affecting memory, word finding, and spatial navigation. In frontotemporal dementia, the proteins tau or TDP-43 spread along the salience network, affecting social conduct, drive, and language, while in Parkinson's disease, alpha-synuclein moves through the brainstem into the cortex, leading to early symptoms related to mood, anxiety, sleep, attention, and movement. When the Lewy body protein has spread from the brainstem to the cortex, a profound dementia can emerge, for which the term "Lewy body dementia" is used. All neurodegenerative conditions eventually affect cognition, psychiatric stability, and movement, but the tempo by which symptoms emerge is the key to diagnosis.

By carefully determining the course of symptoms and the domains that are spared, one can reasonably hypothesize what condition is afflicting the patient. In the case of Cindy's father, the presentation with word-finding difficulty as the first symptom was somewhat atypical for Alzheimer's disease, where problems with memory often predominate early and throughout the course of the illness. Also, a family history helps to determine whether there is a genetic condition that might be responsible for the patient's dementia. The neurological, psychiatric, and motor examinations aid in the refinement of diagnosis. Blood work is done to rule out the treatable causes for dementia, such as low thyroid, vitamin B12 deficiency, or kidney disease. Blood and spinal fluid measures, along with imaging, help to differentiate one dementing condition from another. For example, MRI elucidates the atrophy patterns associated with the different dementias. In Alzheimer's disease (which tends to have memory symptoms), atrophy begins in the hippocampus and posterior portions of the cortex; in frontotemporal dementia (which typically has behavioral or language symptoms), it is in the front part of the brain; and while in parkinsonian disorders (which tend to have more motor symptoms), the atrophy is less distinctive. Vascular conditions are usually visible with MRI, and the less common causes for dementia, such as autoimmune diseases or Jakob-Creutzfeldt disease, have their own unique patterns. Remarkably, now with nuclear imaging (PET scanning), the amyloid protein characteristic of Alzheimer's disease can be visualized. Similarly, the neurofibrillary tangle can be seen with PET. Even more exciting, blood and spinal measures of the Alzheimer, frontotemporal, and parkinsonian proteins are in development and should soon be available to determine diagnosis.

So, diagnosis has come a long way. Today, in good hands, prediction of the underlying genetic and molecular basis for a patient can be reliably determined. If the diagnosis is Alzheimer's disease, treatment with a compound that increases the brain's levels of acetylcholine, a neurotransmitter that is important for attention and memory, is recommended. These medications are not a cure but can stabilize and sometimes improve a patient for as long as one year. If the diagnosis is frontotemporal dementia, medications that treat the mood or behaviors are recommended. With the parkinsonian dementias, acetylcholine-boosting compounds are helpful in diminishing inattention and visual hallucinations. With all of the dementias, it is sometimes necessary to treat sleep, mood, anxiety, and even hallucinations or delusional states with medications. The disease-modifying medications that we all hope for are still just that, a hope. There are multiple pharmaceutical trials focused upon amyloid and tau lowering for Alzheimer's disease, tau- and TDP-43-modifying therapies for the sporadic and familial forms of frontotemporal dementia, and new emerging trials for Parkinson's disease.

Seeing patients and taking their stories is always the highlight of my week. Usually, it is an opportunity to validate a family under stress and to collect their observations. During this time, I think about the intricate way that a neurodegenerative disease intersects with a person's expected trajectory and strengthens or weakens relationships within a family. Finally, the bedside is where I obtain novel insights into the organization of the brain. While the principles underlying decline from a dementia are precise and predictable, taking histories never gets old for me. Every story that I hear is distinctive and enriching. It is, as was said by the narrator from the television show *Naked City*, "There are eight million stories in the naked city. This has been one of them."

A newer generation is pushing for more precise diagnosis using not the history but biomarkers as the basis for diagnosis, and this is a good development, certain to have a real and lasting impact on our society. We will eventually have blood and brain-imaging tests that tell us what neurodegenerative process is present in the brain and help us predict the trajectory for the individual patient. And, there will be treatments for those conditions. With those advances, will my interest in families and their stories become outdated? Maybe, but that was the criticism Frank Benson received, whose research like mine was based upon the collection of stories and tying those stories to the brain.

Biomarkers, a term that is used to describe objective tests that can help with the diagnosis and staging of disease, should supplement, not replace, histories in our relationship with patients and families. We are a social species. Technology will never fully supplant our need to connect, our need to tell and listen to stories and to reflect upon the meaning of those stories. That is who we are. Cindy's story of her father gave me an image of her father's brain in the absence of an MRI. Symptoms began in his early fifties, which meant early onset. Losses in short-term memory indicated a deterioration in the hippocampus, which pointed to Alzheimer's disease. Loss of words for Cindy's dad pointed to the logopenic variant, a language syndrome highly characteristic of Alzheimer's disease. A vulnerability in word finding was the heralding symptom for Jerry.

Since the time Cindy's family sought a diagnosis for Jerry, much has also changed regarding the recognition of the serious burden faced by caregivers and the patient. In many settings, there is a systematic effort to offer support around legal issues like advanced directives, prevention of cardiovascular and psychiatric complications in the patient and caregiver, and finding better ways to support the patient in the home and, when necessary, within nursing facilities. Caregiver burden is substantial with all dementias but varies somewhat depending upon the disease (worse in frontotemporal dementia, where patients become disinhibited and unempathic, rendering them unable to respond to the typical social cues that help to form and maintain relationships) and the hardiness of the caregiver. The Weinstein family was hardy, but some families are broken apart by the appearance of dementia.

We now have better ways of making a diagnosis and supporting caregivers, and these gains will continue. The remaining and more difficult challenge is to translate these sophisticated approaches in diagnosis and care, often available only at academic medical centers, into middle- and low-income communities. The ultimate challenge, still just beyond our reach, will be to use the information that can be derived in diagnosis into powerful disease-modifying and disease-preventing therapies.

• 2 •

Word Finding

Call Me Ahab

Chapter 1 of *Moby-Dick* begins with the iconic sentence "Call me Ishmael." No, the novel actually begins with a list of translations of the word "whale" in a variety of languages, followed by pages and pages of quotations from texts, ranging from the Bible to the songs of sailors, in which the word "whale" appears. Anyway, Ishmael may or may not be the narrator's name. The biblical character of Ishmael, however—lonely, orphaned, wandering—suits the narrator, whose bouts of melancholy result in him following funerals of people he never knew and gravitating toward the beckoning water, which holds the promise of freedom. Ishmael survives his encounter with the water, with Ahab, with Moby Dick, surrounded by the wreckage of death.

For years, my father's death has beckoned me, requiring a reckoning, which is undertaken in this book. I went to his funeral, of course, and even gave a eulogy, but I wasn't really there. It has taken me thirty years to muster the strength to return to the years of his dying and not look away from the wreckage. This year has been a second funeral for my father, but it is actually the first one, because I have been fully present.

• •

After dinner at Dons, you would make me figure
out the tip. If 10% of $10.00 is $1.00, then 5% is
what? My stomach would start churning. I always
hated percentages.

I have a picture of you hugging me — I must be around
5, you close to 40. There's so much love in your eyes, in
your hug, that it almost hurts to look at it.

Your love for me has gotten me through a lot — no,
everything. Geometry, piano lessons, graduate school, your
death. I love thinking of you driving through Essex
Fells, putting the Toyota into 5th gear, being a machine
on the basketball court, taking me to Welsh Farms for
ice cream, wearing your leisure suits, going to Sly and
the family stone with Linda and Lyle, jogging in Verona
Park, our Tuesday nights.

I love remembering these things.
  your delight in getting people to pay their temple dues
  ~~your respect when I told~~
  the first time we went golfing in Inverary and I ended
  up throwing the ball from 1 part of the green to another
  how at every Bar or Bat Mitzvah or wedding, you'd teach
  me how to cha cha or rumba ~~or~~ all over again (and mom, the water
  your ritual of tea and cake after dinner (was never hot enough)
  how angry you got when Pop said to the lawyers that Nana's broken
    hip meant that he couldn't play golf, and he'd never played golf in his life
  how you went to see Grandma on your Bermuda golf trip
  telling me when I hit a wrong note on the piano
  how you'd drive to the Hess gas station to save 3 cents
    per gallon
  setting the timer for long distance calls
  what are we, supporting public service?
  watching Olympic skating with you
  sitting on your lap in the big red chair
  the smell of old spice when you'd hug me or tickle me
  your unconditional love

you've given me so much Dad, been there through
everything even though you haven't been here for a while
your strength has amazed me and often saddened me
in your unwillingness to go gently into that good night
It's over now. Good night I love you.

Cindy's eulogy at Jerry's 1997 funeral

Jerry Weinstein died on August 12, 1997, but was diagnosed with Alzheimer's disease years before. During those years and up until the present (even before he was diagnosed to be honest), *Moby-Dick* has been the book to which I keep returning. How the story of a one-legged captain sailing through the Pacific hunting a whale speaks to me—a Jewish girl from a middle-class family who can't go on boats because of motion sickness—so profoundly is an interesting question whose answer will become clearer in the chapters that follow.

The irony of calling my own chapter "Call Me Ahab" is not lost on me. In fact, irony is a theme that will run throughout these chapters. I am a literary critic, which means that I have devoted most of my life to the study of literature written by authors from Melville to Harriet Beecher Stowe, whom Lincoln is alleged to have said upon their meeting, "So you're the little lady who started this great big war."

Irony is a topic to which I am constitutionally and professionally drawn. We all know ironic people—people who say one thing but mean another—but that's different from irony. Irony is much deeper than an off-the-cuff snarky comment. It is Mark Twain thinking that he is sending Huck Finn and Jim north into freedom and then writing the scene in *Adventures of Huckleberry Finn* where his protagonists get caught in a steamboat accident and miss the turn-off at Cairo (Illinois) and end up going deeper into the South and into slavery. Irony is when Tom Sawyer, in the last third of the novel, makes Jim go through a series of dangerous and pointless acts to escape slavery when Tom knows all along that Jim is free. Irony has a tonal quality of mismatch, which you can read in novels and hear in life. I love the mismatch in novels. It is what I have spent most of my life happily studying. As a rule, I have not liked it very much in life. In fact, I hate it.

Irony is the literary term that perhaps best describes my

twenty-something life in the 1980s. Irony, as I experienced it, was the autobiographical fact of experiencing the best years of one's life at the same time as experiencing the worst. Irony was getting a PhD in the Berkeley English department, or beginning my adult life, at the same time as dealing with (or not dealing with) my father's Alzheimer's diagnosis, or the ending of his life. I'm still not sure which it is or which it was—dealing or not, mine or his—which is, of course, deeply ironic.

Irony is the condition of reading a book a day in preparation for one's oral exams while one of the people you love most in the world—your father—loses (at least) one word a day and can't read a stop sign anymore, and so the car keys must be taken away. Irony is sending weekly letters from the West Coast to the East, knowing full well that the person receiving them can't read, but hoping the act of sending them conveys the deep love that is not just in the words that make up the letters, but in the very fact of those letters existing. The hope that the person receiving them knows that the person writing them is thinking about him and desperately hoping that the receiver can remember just how much he is loved, which is why I often ended the letters with something like, "Always remember that I love you." As if that statement could make it so.

Those letters must have meant something to my dad because one of the last times I went to Florida where my parents lived out the hell that was to become my father's golden years in retirement, I found those letters safely tucked in a drawer in his bedside table in a plastic zip-locked bag. Each letter had been opened so carefully, with the letter opener that my father used to open letters and household bills with (when he could read them) when he was young. He would open the bills that he would always pay on time and then scrupulously balance the checkbook and make sure he would have enough savings that would eventually go to taking care of him in a series of

RYDER'S HOUSE, 1934
Edward Hopper, American, 1882–1967
oil on canvas, 91.6 x 127 cm
Bequest of Henry Ward Ranger through
the National Academy of Design
National Museum of American Art
Smithsonian Institution, Washington, D.C. (1981.76)

WB 60-13689 B

H. GEORGE CASPARI INC.
NEW YORK/ZURICH
Printed in Switzerland

The landlord has a hefty security deposit and I want to get the whole amount back.

Well, I'm going to work on next week's classes. I'll speak with you soon Dad. Give my love to everyone,

Take care and remember I love you.

xx,
Cindy

Dear Dad,   Feb. 13th

Hi there! I just got back from the movies. Mary and I went to see the new Michael J. Fox movie ~~Into the Light~~. It was o.k. Mom said you saw Outrageous Fortune. Wasn't it great? Have you seen the new Woody Allen movie yet? I think I'm going to see Black Widow on Sunday.

So, how are you feeling? Did you have a nice time with Annie + Lenny? How was the gambling boat ride? Did you win any money? Did you get seasick?

Things here are fine. The rainy season has finally begun. The past few days have been rainy + cool. The weathermen say that the rain is good or else there will be a drought this summer. What's the weather like by you? Are you playing much golf? How's the bowling game going?

I'm working pretty hard these days. I wrote a bit this week and hope to write some more this week-end. Thank goodness for the computer. It makes writing 100% easier. This whole process would be much more difficult without the computer.

How's Nana doing? Give her my love when you see her. Have you spoken with Linda recently? Mom told me she's not feeling well. I'm going to try + call her this week-end.

Well Daddy, I'll speak with you soon. Take care and remember I love you.

Love,
Cindy

Two of the letters Cindy wrote to Jerry (years unknown)

expensive and Dantean Florida nursing homes, with each new symptom leading him into a deeper ring of emotional and physical suffering.

Their names were something out of George Orwell's twentieth-century dystopian novel *1984*, in which the Ministry of Truth is a lying factory and the Ministry of Peace is a war machine. The Orwellian world that my dad entered was made up of institutions that included in their names the words "liberty" or "traditions," as if receiving a five-year wheelchair sentence had any relation to liberty, as if the clients of traditions could remember any of them. The nursing homes' relation to language was built on irony, which I realize isn't something a lot of people would necessarily focus on or care much about. But I did, knowing that these words were being used so that the visitors coming in could fool themselves, even for a brief moment, into thinking that they were housing a loved one in something other than a prison. Irony is that this chapter begins with a grandiose claim about the crucial place of *Moby-Dick* in my life and ends with a story about a trip with my dad to a supermarket in Berkeley looking for croutons. A story that isn't really about croutons, as much as it is about the word that designates croutons, and it really isn't about that either. It's about what happens when a mind perpetually can't find words.

• •

The neurological circuitry that explains language acquisition and its demise is incredibly complicated. This observation even applies to the words that explain the deterioration of language. Over lunch at UCSF, a neurologist friend of mine pointed out the irony of this. He said by the time he tells someone that they have early-onset Alzheimer's with the logopenic variant, they have probably lost the word "early." And the logopenic variant isn't the only explanation for a person who can't find words. If a person has frontotemporal dementia and their language is affected, they may have the semantic variant or the nonfluent variant. I remember asking one of the neurologists who specialized in dementia and language how on earth someone could differentiate between these variants, and she said, "Oh, you'll hear it." She was right. I observed a person with the nonfluent variant doing a neuropsychology test in which she was given square tiles, each with a word on it. The task involved arranging the tiles into a sentence that represented the picture. She could not do it because she had lost grammar. The relation between articles, nouns, and verbs went AWOL. Yet another neurologist described this speech as "Tarzan-like."

My dad lost grammar, too, but the first thing he lost was words. He couldn't find them. This is different from the semantic variant, where the meaning of words goes missing. Before Dad lost his words, he knew (I think) what many of them meant, but he could not access them. I witnessed the frustration of this process in a supermarket in Berkeley, where the word "crouton" was just beyond reach. Like a mirage.

There is an idea in literary criticism that describes the relation between the thing that is a crouton and the word that just so happens to designate that crunchy thing in a salad. According to linguist Ferdinand de Saussure, the letters C-R-O-U-T-O-N are marks that comprise what he called the signifier. The signifier, or the sound that those letters make, alludes to the concept, which is the signified, that we have in our minds when we read the word "crouton." The actual thing, or physical object, that we like to eat—the crouton—is the referent. We learn these connections, arbitrary but essential, when we acquire language. We unlearn it when we get Alzheimer's disease. There is no reason on earth why the crunchy thing is called a crouton, but it is.

Some of the books I liked best reveled in this arbitrariness. Take Nathaniel Hawthorne's *The Scarlet Letter* for example. The letter alluded to in the title is an A, and the main character, Hester Prynne, is forced to wear it as punishment for committing adultery with, of all people, the minister of the Puritan church, Arthur Dimmesdale. In the course of the novel, the meaning of the A starts changing. Does the A mean adultery, Arthur, or both or neither? It is all of the above, and even more. Hester embroiders her letter into a gorgeous work of art and transforms her punishment and pain. She transforms her plain A into a badge of honor and of beauty (as a literary critic, I can't help but wonder if A is for aesthetics?). The narrator of the novel even tells us that the Puritan community that had punished Hester with the A comes to think of the A as standing for something good. She is Able. She is an Angel. Hawthorne luxuriates in the plenitude and the richness of language and the many meanings that words, even letters, can convey. Those meanings, Hawthorne reminds us, are made by humans and, therefore, are deeply arbitrary. But who would have thought that when I read *The Scarlet Letter* after my dad's diagnosis, it would fleetingly occur to me, in a moment of being a very bad reader with a predilection for irony taken to an extreme, to mean Alzheimer's? Hester's A was/is not mine, but her project of turning pain into beauty resonates. With Bruce's help, I am trying to find the right words that will translate the mess of grief into the precision and the beauty of language.

My dad was losing himself, and language was—probably because my initial inklings were in long-distance phone calls where his responses to my questions were monosyllabic with no follow-up—the first thing to go, or at least it was the first thing that I fully realized was going. Initially, though, I thought he was "just" depressed. What with selling his business and his house, who wouldn't be?

I imagine that my mother would have a very different perspective on changes in Dad's personality and what Dad lost first, if there were a way of putting into succession those losses. I do not know when other things went—like his ability to balance the checkbook or his confidence behind the wheel—though I learned about many of them from a geographical distance and through the passage of time. Had I been there, I wouldn't have had such a secondary relation to my father's illness, and perhaps wouldn't have had the pileup of relentless guilt that kept me company in Berkeley and hit me like a freight train when he died. But in all likelihood, I probably wouldn't have had a PhD either—oh, or a life.

I do recall one birthday card where Dad's handwriting and spelling were especially atrocious. He never had good handwriting, so it was easy to chalk up his wobbly, malformed letters to carelessness. Looking back, with the benefit of hindsight and a diagnosis, it is clear that he was forgetting how to make letters. The spelling errors, however, gave me pause, and not just because I was getting a degree in English. They were accompanied by a seeming loss of control in the handwriting. The "D" in "Dear" was out of whack, as if a trembling hand were writing it. The "e" dipped below the line of the other letters. There was something different and strange that I was seeing, but it was relatively easy to ignore the wobbly letters and convert the whole thing into a joke about bad penmanship. I didn't think to identify it as a symptom.

I'll talk in the chapters to come about symptoms that couldn't be ignored: my father's loss of direction, the inability to sleep, and the loss of identity that took strangely material forms, like constantly taking his wallet out of his pants pocket to go through it and its forms of identification as if trying to find himself in the documents that named him, but couldn't convey to him what he was really looking for, which was, of course, himself. Let's return to Saussure for a moment. My father had the marks, that is, the letters spelling his name, on the driver's license or the Medicare card, but was searching for what they signified. He couldn't recognize himself. He knew they meant something, but he couldn't figure out what because the referent was under attack. Taking his wallet out and putting it back made him look like a person with an obsessive-compulsive disorder, whose repetitions were without a clear purpose, but he had a purpose. He did, right? And did it help to be reading the symptoms of my dad's illness in this way, seeing or projecting a profundity into what may have been nothing more than a behavioral tic, or was it just my way to intellectualize the horrific reality that my father was disappearing, but still present, without letting myself feel it? A typical English professor would say, it was both. But the ambiguity that I love in novels—the idea that something, whether it is an A, a white whale, the pond in Henry David Thoreau's *Walden*, Walt Whitman's leaves of grass, for example, could mean two or more things at once— wasn't helping. When you read a novel and talk about its ambiguity, the idea isn't to make the ambiguity go away. It's to clarify it. I could be as clear as I wanted to be about the meaning of my dad looking through his wallet, but what I really wanted was for it (the behavior that was a sign of his illness) to go away. My novelistic attempts to deal with the situation only proved that what I wanted was to change my dad's diagnosis, to go back to a time where I would sit on his lap and watch football on Sunday (for God's sake, I loved him so much, I even watched golf and bowling with him), and no amount of interpretation could do that.

One of the most famous quotations attributed to Mark Twain is, "Denial ain't just a river in Egypt." I was in a semi state of denial, ably assisted by none other than Twain and Melville and Hawthorne. I say semi state of denial because, though I knew my father was terribly sick, these beloved authors were like an escape hatch. They helped me temporarily cordon off the threat that was my dad's illness. The threat to him and the threat to me. Novels were like an emergency exit that I could access or a "do not enter" sign that I could put up in order not to fully and directly see the horror of my dad's diagnosis. To do so would have been like looking at Medusa and turning into stone. I should have looked.

But it was devastating watching him take out the wallet scouring it for forms of identification / searching for his identity, put it back, and take it out again. I temporarily recovered from this peek (after all, it was only a peek compared to my mother's perpetual front-row seat) by looking elsewhere—mostly in books. Of course, people look for things all the time, like lost keys or a misplaced article of clothing, but I had never seen someone looking for himself. No matter how many times he looked at his driver's license or Social Security card or Medicare card, the words "Jerry Weinstein" came up short.

This was bad, really bad, but Alzheimer's has a way of setting the bar lower and lower (like limbo, how low can you go?) or more precisely setting the pain quotient higher and higher (here's some more pain—how much can you take?). I should be clear that I'm talking about the person witnessing the person with the disease; that is, myself. It hurts and then you get used to it. And then it hurts some more, and you get used to that. The idea being that with each outrage (a missing memory, a lost word, a trip to the grocery store that ends up taking three hours because the person gets lost and you know this from the odometer), the observer toughens up and prepares for the next onslaught. The narrative of awfulness can be compressed into something like this: first, one takes comfort in the fact that old memories survive even if short ones evaporate; then it's, well he still knows who I am; then it's, at least he knows I'm someone he loves. At a certain point, the idea that "at least he's not dead" becomes laughable. I don't know what my father's narrative of this awfulness would have been.

For me, it was my dad's gradual loss of language—word by word, the drip-drip of language going down the drain—that nearly killed me. It was a torture technique straight out of Greek mythology, like Prometheus getting his liver eaten by a vulture only to have the liver grow back and get eaten again. But if I had to pick the myth that is most applicable, I would say Sisyphus, the king who had to push the boulder up a hill, and it would always fall back down before getting to the top, but with a major caveat. Unlike that Greek king who was greedy and killed people and betrayed his friends, there was no need for my dad to be punished. He was such a good man. He fought in the navy in World War II, loved his kids, worked incredibly hard, and for his efforts got totally screwed. In the early stages of the disease, he was like Sisyphus, except for my dad, the boulder was a word. Unlike Sisyphus, sometimes Dad would get to the top of the hill, and find the word that was waiting there for him, but there was always another word to push up. And at a certain point, like Sisyphus, he would push and not get the word, and the word would come crashing down. And then at another point, he didn't even have the energy to push anymore, and he was smothered by the rocks, by the words that wouldn't move because of the plaques that made mincemeat of his brain.

It was that first iteration of his illness, when words kept slipping through his fingers that made me want to die. Like Hamlet, I wanted to hop in the grave with my dad and never come out. Not that he ever knew about Shakespeare or Hawthorne or Melville, even though he went to Rutgers University on the GI Bill. He never much liked to read even when he could, although now I recall from my youth James Michener's *The Source* (to this day, I have steadfastly refused to read it) sitting on his impeccably kept night table—the one with his worn-in slippers perfectly arranged underneath—month after month, year after year. I wonder if long ago, he started having trouble reading. Or maybe he preferred Leon Uris (I can still see his tattered, blue-covered copy of *Exodus*) to Michener.

Having refused to read Michener in some weird statement of daughterly solidarity, I would venture to guess that the only thing that he and Melville have in common is that both wrote long books and their last names began with M. *Moby-Dick* is the novel probably most interested in and successful at demonstrating language's breadth and beauty. The novel is so inextricably a part of our cultural DNA that even if a person hasn't read the book, just about everyone knows that the story is about a one-legged captain, named Ahab, who is in charge of a New England whale ship called the *Pequod* and who understands human nature so well (except his own) that he manages to get the sailors on the ship to identify so deeply with his pain at having his leg (et al.) eaten by this one white whale that they'll devote their time and their lives to the fulfillment of his vengeance. Along the way, the crewmembers kill many other whales and so the economic component of the hunt is satisfied. Ahab charms the crew or, perhaps more accurately, hypnotizes them by his language, which is a combination of Shakespeare meets the God of the Old Testament. Ahab is mesmerizing, and he mesmerizes through his language, and there are lots of images in the novel that refer to Ahab's magnetic personality and godlike powers. The reader is NOT, I repeat NOT, supposed to identify with Ahab.

That pride of place is reserved for Ishmael. Ishmael is the character with whom the reader is meant to connect. He is funny, open-minded—as evidenced by his physical and mental acceptance of the capaciously tattooed Queequeg—and not a sore loser (he is at the bottom of the totem pole when it comes to how much each of the sailors will earn upon their return to New England, but doesn't really care). Ishmael is the sailor who finds his way to the *Pequod* because he is a depressed sort who looks for comfort offshore. Because he is the only member of the crew to make it out alive, he tells the story, though at times there is a kind of tug-of-war for narrative space between Ishmael and Ahab. His presence in the novel competes with Ahab's, and their storylines intersect and diverge. Intersect because Ahab is Ishmael's captain, and at times Ishmael does seem to be seduced by the brute and eloquent force of Ahab's hatred of the whale, and diverge because Ishmael is also constantly upending Ahab's approach to the world. Whereas Ahab sees only himself and his pain in virtually every aspect of the world ("Ahab is Ahab"), Ishmael is devoted to capturing every aspect of the world that is not himself. Ahab is the narcissist. Ishmael is the opposite. Ahab's universe closes in upon itself and himself. Ishmael's moves outward in his enormous embrace of difference and multiplicity. He is anthropologist, scientist, lawyer, sailor, humorist, and student. "The whale ship was my Yale College and my Harvard," he memorably notes.

Ishmael's hold on the reader is much more intellectual than Ahab's, and therefore more fragile. His language is a tour de force of literary (not just Old Testament and Shakespearean tragic heroes), scientific, and global references. While Ahab is busy coming up with ways to kill the whale, Ishmael spends his time describing the whale in ways that make it more human. He seems to know (or at least want to know) everything about the whale—whether he is telling us about the whale's skin, skeleton, or head—despite the fact that so many of his chapters are about how we can ultimately know very little about the whale. One of my favorite chapters is when Ishmael talks about trying to figure out what the heck is coming out of the whale's spout. He has various theories, which all must remain untested because to really know what that gas/liquid is, Ishmael would have to put his face so close to the spout that he would in all likelihood be terribly scalded or perish in finding out the answer. The importance of Ishmael's chapters is not the end result, but the process of getting there. In other words, the chapters frequently end with our having zero knowledge about some detail about the whale, but the knowledge we gain is in Ishmael's description of trying and failing to acquire some specific factoid. We may not ultimately learn what the stuff is spurting out of the whale's head, but we occupy an intelligence that is insatiably curious, and the language that is produced out of that sense of wonderment is beautiful, risible, and itself full of wonder.

Literary critics read their favorite books many times over, and I have read *Moby-Dick* many times. The first time was when I was sixteen, and I dutifully tracked the biblical allusions in the novel in order to explain how Melville was using and revising the Bible in order to tell this story of a man who hated God so much that one could only conclude that at some point in time, he loved God so much that he felt like a jilted lover. Ahab responded with a God-defying, self-destructive vengeance that also destroyed everyone else in his path, with the exception of Ishmael. In college, I read *Moby-Dick* again in a sophomore-year seminar taught by a teacher who would become my beloved academic father, and in that paper, I talked about the conflict in the novel between Ahab's penchant for allegorical certainty (the whale is evil and therefore must be destroyed) and Ishmael's embrace of symbolic potentiality (the whale is destructive, sublime, unknowable, domestic, feral, and a bunch of other things, too). I would revise this account of allegory in my dissertation for graduate school, and it would become the basis of my first book.

That would happen, however, only after reading *Moby-Dick* for a senior thesis with that same beloved teacher, to whom I proudly remarked that I was reading the novel for the third time, and he replied, "Well, maybe now you'll have something to say about it." With those words, I was completely taken with this professor, and obviously with Melville, and found myself reading *Moby-Dick* again in my first year of graduate school with a different and also beloved professor. He would tell me, once I had my father's diagnosis and finally knew why my phone calls with him were so short and strange and unsatisfying, that if I left Berkeley for a graduate program on the East Coast (I was thinking Johns Hopkins) and thought I could commute from Maryland to Florida to help my mother take care of my father, I should just forget it. Either stay in Berkeley and do the PhD or move to Florida and be with my parents. I couldn't have it both ways. I would do a crummy job with both if I tried. He was right, but man was I in trouble. Not nearly as much as my father, of course, but I heard a small bell in my brain sounding the alarm. The poet Emily Dickinson wrote, "I felt a Funeral, in my Brain." Me too. This was a choice from which I might never quite recover. That has turned out to be true.

• •

I read *Moby-Dick* again shortly after my father was diagnosed and had a very different experience of the novel. Prior to that, when I was in my right mind, relatively speaking, I identified with Ishmael. I got his humor (he describes the whale's phallus, the outer portion of which he compares to the Pope donning his robes) and loved his subversion of authority (take that Ahab!). Most of all, I reveled in his wordplay, his gorgeous prose, and the fascinating associations between whaling and writing or between the history of whaling and the history of the world. For instance, Ishmael's chapter about the whale's skin begins with a description of its texture and transparency and ends up linking the whale's skin to a fragile piece of paper. When I teach *Moby-Dick*, one of the things I like to do most is guide bewildered students through a particularly dense passage where Ishmael takes the reader's hand and walks through global history, by linking one place or one image to another, in one paragraph.

It is probably a good thing that during my oral examination none of my questioners pressed me too hard on *Moby-Dick* because when I reread it after having learned that my dad had Alzheimer's, my interpretive radar was all wrong. It was like the compasses on the *Pequod* going haywire. I felt like Pip, the character who falls out of one of the boats while the crew is chasing a whale and gets hurled into the middle of the ocean. While the crew is deciding whether or not to save him, he is forced to endure several minutes immersed in the enormity of the Pacific Ocean during which time he contemplates death, sees God, and goes mad. Pip is eventually rescued and befriended by Ahab, and with friends like that, I was clearly in trouble. My (mis)reading of the novel made the problem clear to me. Ishmael no longer seemed very funny or even very relevant to the plot of the novel. I knew that was wrong, interpretively speaking, but in my new frame of mind and with my revised frame of reference, it was all about Ahab, his pain, his insatiable desire for revenge, the hunt. I understood that terrible and insane character in a way I never had before and hopefully never will again. His rage was my rage. Like him, someone had taken something, someone very close to me, and I was angrier and sadder than I had ever been in my life. I never believed in God so, in a key departure from Ahab, anger at God wasn't the problem. Rather, I had always believed in family and the love of family, more specifically my father, and the love of my father for me, which was so true and so deep that it even lasted until he had no idea who I was, couldn't speak, and was medicated out of his mind (he had been out of his mind, but I hope being stoned made that somewhat easier). I say he loved me, but really what I mean is that I think, on some level, he remembered that I was someone he had loved. Even if he didn't know exactly who I was, he knew I was someone who had mattered to him once upon a time.

If someone remembers having loved you, is that the same as them loving you? Not exactly, but close enough. I could work with that because it meant that there was enough of my dad there, which meant I was there too. It's a funny thing—no, more like devastating—when someone who knows you doesn't know you anymore. It makes you feel, it made me feel that I was disappearing too. I ended up persuading myself, even if it were a fiction, that, as spectral as my dad had become, he still loved me, remembered having loved me, and so I still existed. A gossamer, but essential acknowledgment—my sense that there was a memory of a former acknowledgment—would suffice. I could survive, as his daughter, with this much or this little. It allowed me to do what literary critics do and find meaning (and, as his daughter, preserve his love for me). I could create a narrative out of bits and pieces. I just needed to get off the surface of my dad (his mouth open, his shaky gait—when he could still walk—his stare) and look deeper.

Being a literary critic came to my rescue. It might seem that *Moby-Dick* is only about a whale, but it is also about God, pain, language, economics, slavery. Similarly, the student of literature advised the daughter, it might seem that your dad has no idea who you are, but if you look more closely, you'll find meaning, and when you find that, you'll find your dad's love for you and you'll find him. Looking back, I think this psychic position was both a problem and not a problem (maybe I can hold two ideas in my mind now, but I couldn't then): a problem in that it kept my dad's illness at bay, preventing me from really "dealing" with it, and not a problem, allowing me to keep my dad's illness at bay and permitting me to do the work I loved. Dealing with it this way (or is this not dealing with it?), that is, by adopting a crouch position like a child afraid of looking under the bed for fear of finding something really scary (my dad always told me I was a fraidy-cat, and boy, he didn't know the half of it), allowed me to have the life that I wanted ever since I was sixteen and read *Moby-Dick* for the first time and thought, this is what I want to do forever. But how could any self-respecting daughter who loved her father do what she wanted to when he was disappearing? How could I do anything at all, let alone be happy doing it, when my dad couldn't do anything?

And as I reread *Moby-Dick* for the umpteenth time, with my dad's illness firmly in place, even if only on the margins of my consciousness (reading provided relief, putting Alzheimer's to the side while I tried to make sense of the novel), Ahab's soliloquy about piling on the hump of the whale all of the pain and sadness of human existence nevertheless hit the nail right on my head. The insanity of locating one's pain in one place in order to kill it once and for all seemed not only perfectly logical but also eminently possible. If only there were a white whale that I could find and kill, I'd feel way better. For a while, I thought Florida was the answer. I never liked Florida all that much, except for the times my mom and I would visit Grandma Sarah in Miami Beach, and now that it was the site where my father was living out this nightmare, my feelings about the state went even further south.

But maybe the white whale was hiding somewhere in Berkeley. In my orals list? A leviathan of sorts comprised of hundreds of books that I could make my way through and destroy. I totally slayed my orals, which made me happy for a short while, but it wasn't as satisfying as finding the thing that was the source of my pain (and my dad's) and destroying it. The

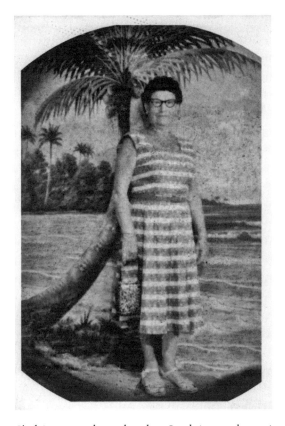

Cindy's maternal grandmother, Sarah (year unknown)

problem was that I loved the books I read. Even the ones I hated I loved. Frank Norris, a writer in the late nineteenth century, who, coincidentally enough, spent some time at Berkeley, wrote a novel called *McTeague* that I endlessly made fun of by calling it McTedious. *An American Tragedy*, written by Theodore Dreiser in 1925 and turned into the 1951 film *A Place in the Sun*, which starred Elizabeth Taylor, Montgomery Clift, and Shelley Winters, was over nine hundred pages, and as much as the title resonated with what I felt my family was going through, the story of Clyde Griffiths's downfall, the protagonist who ends up put to death in an electric chair, was riveting. Reading close to a book a day both kept my pain at arm's length and allowed me to read about other people's (I mean characters') pain, so mine didn't hurt quite so much.

All of which is to say, I couldn't find anything resembling a white whale in Berkeley. The city was too beautiful. The bookstores were too seductive. The cafes were too ubiquitous. A friend of mine used to say, "Coffee makes you smarter." If that were true, we were all on the road to winning a Nobel Prize. Berkeley was clearly where I was meant to be. I was happy, despite the fact that every night when I went to bed after spending the day studying and not thinking about my dad, the heaviness in my heart came back, and I couldn't take a deep breath. My happiness was the perfect double-edged sword.

There are many moments in *Moby-Dick* that have served as touchstones in my life. One is the image of the nursing female whales circling around their baby whale children. This is important because there are so few females in the novel, other than Aunt Rachel who brings food aboard the *Pequod* before it launches. It is also important because the chapter offers a picture of serenity amidst many other chapters where whales are being hunted and dismembered. Another is when Ahab addresses the whale in the chapter called "The Sphynx," and asks the head, which is attached to the side of the *Pequod*, to disclose its secrets, such as what things the whale has seen in its watery travels and whether or not there is a God. Another image that haunts me from the novel is the sailors who create representations—in images and texts—of the physical and emotional damage endured by a life at sea. A missing arm. A capsized boat and a drowning fellow sailor. They have these representations with them at all times as they stand, if they're lucky, or sit and beg with their bodies wounded, waiting for passersby to have mercy on them and spare them a dime.

I think this book that I am writing is that for me—me, the person decimated by my father's disappearing act that he never agreed to and that I never gave my permission for (as if anyone asked). Or maybe this is the book that I write for my dad, had he been able to read, write, speak. This would be his representation of his pain, or it is at least my attempt to speak for him. We all know that a person in pain who can't speak is in even more pain. That's why people have "do not resuscitate" orders. I heard the pain of my dad's Alzheimer's disease in the cries, whimpers, and the half-spoken words that stopped midstream because the words, like the person trying to utter them, lost direction. I saw the hole in the wall where the sink was in the nursing home where he was to spend the last years of his life, but the sink was no longer there because my father pulled it out in a fit of rage. I, maybe you, could feel it in the lips that desperately try to put themselves together to make a kiss, but can't and instead touch the skin on your cheek as if knowing there is more to be done, but no longer knowing how to. Unlike those wounded sailors, though, I'm not looking for a dime or anything like that. I'm looking to spare myself.

There is another moment from *Moby-Dick* that strikes me as equally germane to this enterprise of writing this book and reckoning with my father's illness and the years spent not being there to fend it off, as if I could have, or not being there to take care of him, which I could have. That image is in the chapter called "The Sperm-Whale's Head." Ishmael talks about the placement of the whale's eyes. He first describes the strange fact that the whale's eyes are located where human ears are found, and then reflects upon the optical and hermeneutic, or interpretive, implications of this anomalous placement. Optically, this means that a whale can hold in its brain two completely different images at the same time. One eye might see a sea of brit, one of the whale's main sources of food.

The other eye might see a shiver of sharks. Conceptually, the point is that one mind, the whale's mind, can apprehend two images—perhaps even contradictory ones—at once. For Melville, this becomes a profound lesson in how we read literature and how we understand life. The idea is actually quite simple in theory, and hard as hell in practice. Ishmael gets this. Ahab does not. The whale's ability to see two pictures simultaneously exemplifies an ideal of human perception and open-mindedness; that the world and one's life are made up of multiple and often mutually exclusive experiences. The whiteness of the whale, that is Moby Dick, might signify the purity of an angel or the terror of dead bones. If one could see two things at once, one might envision, on the one hand, a beautiful day, and on the other hand, a homeless person struggling to get through that day. One might be able to hold the joyful experience of being in Berkeley and doing the thing I had always wanted to do—to read—while knowing that my father was somewhere in Florida, perhaps lost, frightened that pieces of him were falling off, and he couldn't find them anywhere. Let alone read.

In my head, I wanted to be the whale and keep these two equally true experiences in my mind at once, but in my heart, I couldn't help but compartmentalize and pick one. Because my dad's illness felt much more real and important than my life as a graduate student, I picked my dad (sort of), even though I stayed in Berkeley. So I guess I also picked Berkeley. Over the years, I would do an excellent job of punishing myself for trying to have it both ways—of attempting to put into human practice what the whale did by simply being a whale. Actually, what I did was I divided my time (and perspective) in two. By day, happy graduate student. By night, devastated daughter. I couldn't hold the two in my mind at the same time.

Such a compartmentalizing approach, what today might best

be described as a dangerous absence of mindfulness, yielded success on the academic battlefront. And that's because it wasn't a battlefront at all. When my head was in a book, I was out of the line of fire. My mind was elsewhere—at Walden Pond with Thoreau or on the Mississippi River with Huck and Jim. Anywhere but in that godforsaken nursing home with the melody of irony coursing through its musical repertoire—I remember being overcome by a feeling of nausea when the song "Thanks for the Memories" was the nursing home's background music—and the ghostly people in their wheelchairs, mouths agog, waiting to get off of death row, by which I mean actually, finally die. Sure, it was challenging trying to make sense of Melville's fifth novel, *Mardi*, the one he wrote as a kind of (failed) dress rehearsal for *Moby-Dick*, but it was peace, or rather it was Melville's struggle. I settled into writing my thesis as if covering myself with a warm blanket. I was under the counterpane, the blanket shared by Ishmael and Queequeg in the Spouter Inn before they sign up to work on the *Pequod*, with them. My work was my salvation. Find a job? No problem. Prepare for the interview? Bring it on. Get the book published and go through the tenure process. Harder, much harder.

But still, compared to some of my more memorable episodes with Dad, everything related to work was a dream come true. If I weren't trying to show my dad how to put film into a camera that he once used to love taking pictures with, it was easy. If I weren't explaining to him how to cut a cantaloupe, it was grand. If I weren't lying to him about the fact that he had Alzheimer's disease—my mother had put a gag order on all of us—and being commanded to respond to his frightened inquiries about why he was forgetting things with, "Everyone forgets," it was heaven. My mother intoned, "Don't tell him. He'll kill himself." And he would have, which is why I have a backup plan. In case my loved ones get all sentimental on me and think that just because I seem to recognize them once a week I should stay alive, I have asked a friend, who has promised me that she will prevail and make sure my wishes are respected, to pull the plug, push me off a cliff, take me to Amsterdam, whatever.

I think some of my difficulty stemmed from the fact that truth and fiction were in a knot that I couldn't untangle. I was being told to make up a story that my dad wouldn't know was a story. So visit after visit, while he was being invaded by this disease, I would sit next to my dad in Dunkin' Donuts in West Palm Beach and hear him talk about how sad he was that he couldn't remember things that happened yesterday (this was when he could still speak), and I would reply that his memory of the more important things—the things in his deeper past— was still solid. In telling him this, I was obviously trying to convince myself, too. It was all bullshit, though. He knew it, I'm certain, but was desperate to feel comforted, so he didn't "let on," to use a favorite phrase of Huck Finn's, that he knew it was all crap. I was creating this fiction for my dad, and he was believing it, sort of, when what I really wanted to do was tell him the truth so he could take it from there (if he could remember the truth long enough and what he had always said he wanted to do in the face of it). Thus, by honoring my mother's wishes, I was totally dishonoring my father's. The one conversation that I really wanted to have with my dad, the one where I tell him how terribly, sickeningly sorry and crushed and annihilated I was that he was losing his mind and how could I help him end his life, if that is what he still wanted to do, I couldn't have. I'm having it now because even though it's too late and kind of pointless from the point of view of changing anything, it's the best I can do. I'm having it now in what is at once a kind of soliloquy, because my dad is the one I speak to and write for. It is also a dialogue, both with Bruce, who can use the language of science to describe my father's symptoms for those readers for whom references to Melville only go so far, and with readers for whom these psychic gymnastics may serve as a warning or as a guide (or both?).

There were other conversations I didn't have but wish I could have. They weren't as necessary as the one I wanted to have with my dad, but they would have been good to have nonetheless. One would have been to beg my mom to give me permission to tell my dad exactly what disease he had. Actually, by the time my dad was given the diagnosis, and we were allowed to say the A word, it didn't matter because he couldn't hold it. I wish I had talked with the doctors who diagnosed my father and who cared for him (if you can call writing out endless numbers of prescriptions "care") as opposed to sitting in doctor offices listening carefully to everything, but feeling like I was in the midst of "the big one"; that is, the earthquake that every geologist tells us is only a matter of time. During an earthquake, you're supposed to duck and cover, which is what I did. I didn't hide under a table. I hid in books. I have sort of forgiven myself that as the twenty-five-year-old I was, I was too young to engage, too afraid to ask the questions about what was coming down the pike lest I get run over. There wasn't a seat belt that could keep me from dying in the emotional car crash that I was certain would be the cost of having a head-on collision with my dad's disease.

I thought I didn't crash—after all, I got a PhD—but I did. The collision wasn't exactly head-on, but it was bad and, of course, unavoidable. It happened when my father at long last died, and I nearly died too—of sadness, of guilt, of things not said. For several years, novels were a kind of seat belt for me, but they were fictional, and if a seat belt is fiction, is it real? This book is my chance to understand not how to get it right this time because that's impossible, but it's my best shot at making sense of the road I was on—mine, not Jack Kerouac's—where fiction and reality merged, switched places, illuminated things, shrouded others.

• •

I think I was dreaming in Berkeley and only woke up to reality when I was with my dad (and then finally when I wasn't). Case in point: going with him to a supermarket in Berkeley on one of his and my mom's last visits to California. This visit was the first time that I witnessed my dad not knowing who my mom was. When we walked to the supermarket, he asked me with a combination of fright and curiosity, who is that woman in the house? Being asked this question by my father made writing two pages a day, which is what I did to get my dissertation done, feel like a piece of cake.

It was a beautiful spring day in Berkeley, and that evening, we were going to make dinner at my house. Dad wanted a salad with his chicken. This seemed like a rather straightforward proposition until we got closer to the market, and Dad realized he wanted something very specific in his salad but couldn't remember what it was. I was always good with words, having been trained in the arts of playing Scrabble at a very young age with a very competitive mother, and then spending hours on the *New York Times* crossword puzzle as a college student (pre-Google). I was therefore confident that I could help Dad get to the right word with little fuss. Cocky, rational me went into problem-solving mode. Initially, I thought he wanted a certain kind of lettuce and not just iceberg. We were in Berkeley after all, and Dad had succumbed to the charms of the gourmet ghetto with its gorgeous produce and cheese varieties. Arugula? No. Red Leaf? No. He made it clear that it wasn't lettuce that he wanted, but it was something in the salad. Goat cheese? No. Tomatoes? No. Chickpeas? No. Sprouts? No.

I was starting to get a little antsy myself as I realized I wasn't hitting my mark. Dad picked up his pace as if speed would help him find the word more quickly, as if the word were running away from him and walking faster would help him catch it. I suggested that we might be able to figure out what it was that he wanted once we got to the market, and we could go through the aisles. Use your Saussure. Find the visible referent in the absence of having the signifier (at this point, Dad had the signified). That calmed him (and me) down for a bit, and then we entered the market. For some reason, I was set on the idea that it was chickpeas that he wanted, but he just wasn't connecting the word to the thing. Thus, I gently directed us toward the beans. Bad move. He got angry not only because he didn't want chickpeas, but also because he realized that I was behaving as if I thought he didn't know what the word "chickpea" referred to. He was right to be angry, and I was right to treat him like a child because he was one, sort of. I now see his anger as a good thing—he was angry that I was treating him like a child, and he was healthy enough to know it. As the disease progressed, I came to miss that anger because it had confirmed for me that some structures remained in place. He was still my father and I his child. Absent the anger, that was gone. He was gone, too, and so was I.

I regrouped us, and we walked toward the produce aisle. He told me it wasn't anything like that, as in nothing refrigerated. What the fuck was it? Capers? I didn't think he liked capers, but the past was pretty irrelevant as I also thought he knew the woman to whom he had been married for over thirty years. At a certain point, my dad's desperation became my own. I couldn't find the word, the thing—who cared which? Saussure wasn't helping. No longer were we walking through the various aisles, which was another one of my initial strategies (saunter through the aisle and maybe he'll see what he wants and that will be that), considering other things we might have wanted with dinner. It was all about finding whatever it was that we were looking for. Our white whale. Who knew it was croutons?

The two of us began a frantic search through the aisles. With fear and hope, I watched my dad looking at the various cans and boxes of stuff on the shelves, his expression turning from hope to disappointment to sadness and back again with each swift rejection of not seeing the thing he could not name. I decided it would be worse for me to keep guessing, so I shut my mouth and just kept him company on his heartbreaking journey through the supermarket. Eventually, we found the croutons. Dad's face lit up. He was so incredibly happy; I could have cried for joy myself. It was over. The relief was physical. Our hunt through the oceans of salad paraphernalia was over. We could go home, make the damned salad, and eat.

Until my dad decided that he wanted to rent a movie. I'll cut to the chase and tell you it was *Ferris Bueller's Day Off*. But my dad didn't, couldn't find the words. And so we started all over again.

Where Dementia Decides to Dance

A crouton is a small, square-shaped piece of fried bread that is placed into soups or salads. The crouton originated in France in the 1800s, where a rich and complex food culture was emerging, and humans were creating a new way of cooking and eating. Croutons are an acquired taste, rarely appreciated by young children, but by early adulthood many of us begin to enjoy the aesthetic of eating a soft and chewy green salad with dressing that is dotted with hard and crunchy croutons. The actual origin of "crouton" is from the Latin word *crout*, which signifies crust. As is often the case with the English language, simply following phonetic rules does not help us to spell "crouton." Rather, we associate the orthograph—the written constellation of letters—with the meaning for the word, which allows us to remember the correct pronunciation. Most of us infrequently eat, speak about, or write, the word "crouton." It is a word that is used with low frequency by most people. Unless, of course, we are cooks and place croutons in salads every day or fanatically eat salads with croutons on a daily basis.

Ordinarily, words that we use frequently, like mother, father, shirt, cup, table, or house, are more facilely produced than a word like crouton. Therefore, it is not surprising that Jerry Weinstein, as part of his inability to name items (anomia) had difficulty generating "crouton" during a conversation with his daughter. Jerry's struggle to remember "crouton" is the first moment that Cindy becomes aware that he is having cognitive issues. Anomia is one of the earliest manifestations of Jerry's Alzheimer's disease. Soon afterward, Cindy realizes that there are other signs of trouble. Jerry was never much of a reader, but now his spelling is off, and his writing is shaky. How disturbing for Cindy, a voracious reader, writer, and emerging literary critic, to see her father struggle to name, spell, or write. A steady cascade of losses soon follows, and, like many, Cindy watches her beloved parent descend into the dementia of Alzheimer's disease.

Notably, his first symptoms are in the domain of language. The language form of Alzheimer's disease that begins with anomia is called logopenic aphasia, or the logopenic variant of primary progressive aphasia. This Latin phrase, *logopenic aphasia*, is loosely translated as a paucity of words. Logopenic aphasia was first described by my colleague Marilu Gorno Tempini at UCSF in 2004, and it is characterized by anomia (inability to name), loss of reading, or alexia, and loss of writing, or agraphia. Scientists are just beginning to understand these deficits, and the findings hold unexpected implications about how our brains work and how this influences the sorts of disorders to which we are vulnerable.

The Three Variants of Dementia That Begin in Language Regions

Where in the brain the dementia decides to dance determines the symptoms and deficits that we exhibit. In addition to the logopenic variant of Alzheimer's disease, there are two other dementia sub-types that begin in language regions and start clinically as a language disorder—nonfluent variant primary progressive aphasia and semantic variant primary progressive aphasia. Like the logopenic variant, these dementia subtypes begin in the left hemisphere and start as a disorder of language. Study of these distinctive forms of what is called primary progressive aphasia has informed linguists, neuroscientists, and clinicians about the organization of language in the brain and the selective vulnerability of different brain regions to different subtypes of dementia.

First, let me explain what these progressive aphasias have taught us about language. The nonfluent variant was less mysterious and uncharted than the semantic variant, because the nonfluent variant hit a region in the brain that is vulnerable to stroke, the left fronto-opercular region. In 1863, Paul Broca described aphasia associated with injury to this region in the setting of stroke, and the scientific community has had 150 years to study Broca's aphasia. The clinical features of nonfluent variant primary progressive aphasia are largely indistinguishable from patients with Broca's aphasia due to stroke. Broca's region, the left fronto-opercular area, is a language area responsible for the fluent output of speech, and with the non-fluent syndrome, a person says fewer words, phrases get shorter, and there is increased effort in getting words out (sputtering, extra gesticulation), along with problems understanding and generating correct grammar. Otherwise, comprehension is relatively intact. Abnormalities occur in morphology (verb tense) and in syntax (word order) which are called morphosyntactic errors. A typical example is when someone attempts to say, "I went to the store," but she takes thirty seconds to sputter out, "I store goed."

**MAIN DIFFERENCES AMONG THE THREE VARIANTS
OF PRIMARY PROGRESSIVE APHASIA**

	Semantic Variant Primary Progressive Aphasia	Nonfluent Variant Primary Progressive Aphasia	Logopenic Variant Primary Progressive Aphasia
Clinical Diagnosis	• Impaired naming • Impaired single-word meaning: "Bird, what is a bird?" • Surface dyslexia or dysgraphia: "Yacht" is spelled "Yot" • Spared speech production (grammar is normal)	• Fewer words • Agrammatism: "I there goed" • Effortful, halting speech with gesticulations and hand movement • Spared single-word comprehension • Normal comprehension	• Word-finding pauses in spontaneous speech: "I was looking for my . . . my . . . um keys" • Impaired repetition of sentences and phrases • Spared single-word comprehension • Spared motor speech (no distortions) • Absence of frank agrammatism
Atrophy on MRI	 svPPA Predominant anterior temporal lobe	 nfvPPA Predominant left posterior-fronto-insular	 lvPPA Predominant left posterior perisylvian or parietal

Source: Images from Zachary A. Miller, Maria Luisa Mandelli, Katherine P. Rankin, et al., "Handedness and Language Learning Disability Differentially Distribute in Progressive Aphasia Variants," *Brain*. 2013;136/11,3461–73, by permission of Oxford University Press.

By contrast, the semantic variant of primary progressive aphasia described by Arnold Pick in 1892 in his original cases is distinctive and novel. It was ignored until the primary progressive aphasias were rediscovered in the 1990s by Marsel Mesulam. Unlike the nonfluent variant, the semantic variant was not seen with stroke and was novel when it was presented to the medical, language, and neuroscience communities. Unlike the areas involved in the logopenic variant (posterior temporal parietal) and the nonfluent variant, which are commonly hit by strokes, the semantic variant is caused by dysfunction in the anterior temporal lobes, a region rarely involved with strokes.

From the study of this disorder, an important and unique role for the anterior temporal lobes in language was discovered. With the semantic variant, people lose words and lose the meaning of words. Unlike Jerry, who had trouble pulling the word "crouton" out of his left posterior temporal-parietal region but once it was said, was able to recognize it perfectly, someone with semantic variant loses the richly layered content and meaning associated with a word like crouton. If Jerry had semantic variant, when the word "crouton" was offered by Cindy, Jerry would likely have countered, "Crouton? What is a crouton?" So, this is more than just a naming deficit. Rather, semantic variant strips someone of their world constructs, their understanding of what things are. While all of us know what a dog is, when we ask a person with semantic variant to draw a dog, it has features of multiple animals, as the concept of dog becomes blurred. Eventually, the individual with semantic variant loses knowledge about all items and lives in a world without concepts that are language-based.

While the logopenic aphasia nearly always predicts Alzheimer's disease, the nonfluent variant predicts frontotemporal dementia associated with aggregation of the tau protein. Semantic variant is also associated with frontotemporal dementia, but the molecule underlying this language subtype is TDP-43, not tau. So, we have three different language subtypes that cause three different types of deficits in language, hit three different regions of the cortex on the left side of the brain, and are all caused by different molecules. This is the wonder of what neurologists call neuronal specificity. Each disease starts in a specific region, with the different regions selectively vulnerable to different molecules. This remarkable and mysterious story is one of the topics that continues to fascinate those of us who study these focal neurodegenerative conditions.

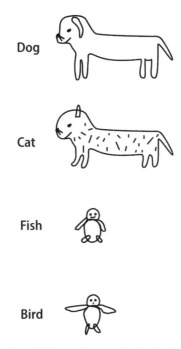

An example of the loss of semantic details. The animals
all start to look alike and have only rudimentary
characteristics specific to their genus (if they have them
at all). Illustration typical of numerous patient files.
Drawing by Caroline Prioleau

The Wonder of Language

No domain in the brain garners as much respect as language. We
learn to speak, read, and write as children due to uniquely human
capacities of the brain, and we carry these skills with us to our grave,
unless as with Cindy's father, neurodegenerative disease, a stroke,
or another catastrophic brain injury intervenes. For right-handers,
the left side of the brain is highly specialized for language—written, read, and spoken—a pattern that is set in the third trimester
in utero, when neurons are migrating and dividing, and the brain

is still being formed. Conversely, the right side of the brain is specialized for visual tasks, such as painting, carpentry, or mechanical skills, and for social skills and behaviors. Most left-handers also have left-brain specialization for language, although in approximately 40 percent, language is localized predominantly on the right side. For most of us, and nearly all right-handers, the left side of the brain is poised to speak when we are born. Yet, if as an infant or as a young child, we are raised in isolation and are not exposed to language, even with extensive tutoring, our language comprehension and output will remain abnormal throughout life. The first years of life are a critical period for language, and if the circuits that we are born with aren't stimulated, they never work quite right. Susan Curtis, a brilliant linguist at UCLA, has noted that children brought up without language for more than a few years are profoundly and permanently impaired in language, even when they are resocialized. The left side of the brain is wired at birth to name, read, and write. Yet, these innately wired abilities will develop only if the environment is right and we take advantage of this uniquely human wiring.

In socially and economically developed societies, most of us start reading by five or six years of age, and we are proficient readers by the time we are teenagers. And what a remarkable gift and advantage we have when we learn to read and write. The deep and rich world that is opened up by reading, writing, and learning new words accounts for many unique aspects of our humanity. Our closest living relative, the chimpanzee, which separated from the human line during evolution more than seven million years ago, has minimal spoken and no written language. Written language, which appeared just five thousand years ago, offers us the ability to read the thoughts and observations of others, to learn about new mysterious words and worlds, and to self-reflect about who we are. Reading is strongly linked to writing and naming, and doing one enhances the other. And all of these functions are localized to left posterior temporal-parietal brain circuits.

When I began to read, my grandfather Herman, an intellectual and an Anglophile, introduced me to *Tom Brown's School Days*, a book by Thomas Hughes about a private school in England. Published in 1872, the book explored the life and adventures set in nineteenth-century Victorian England, emphasizing strong principles about bullying, courage, honor, and fairness, all learned in a private school for boys during this time. This world is largely gone, but it was one that intrigued me as a young boy living in a very different world of suburban midwestern America. It started with my grandfather reading to me in the evening, but soon I learned to read independently and cherished this first book given to me by Grandpa Herman, which I reread many times. After a reading, as I drifted to sleep, I imagined living in this ancient world, blending my own adventures with this world that I had never really known. *Tom Brown's School Days* left an indelible mark on my consciousness that created a world that was as real, even more real, than my own experiences in Madison, Wisconsin. I became a bibliophile and by the time I had finished junior high school, I had read Henry Fielding's *Tom Jones*, William Golding's *Lord of the Flies*, and *Adventures of Huckleberry Finn* by Mark Twain. These books reinforced principles that I learned from Tom Brown and also left me with new ones. My family was minimally religious, but reading the books of Saul Bellow, Philip Roth, and Bernard Malamud in high school exposed me to a post–World War II urban Jewish consciousness that was intriguing. College brought me challenging novels, such as *Ulysses*, by James Joyce, *Been Down So Long It Looks Like Up to Me*, by Richard Fariña, and *Gravity's Rainbow*, by Thomas Pynchon. In fact, it was *Gravity's Rainbow* that stimulated my first interest in science.

Reading served me well in life, transforming and enriching my thinking and leaving me with a rigor around the English language. When I decided to study medicine after completing college, I learned new epistemologies and approximately ten thousand new words. Training in neurology brought new ideas and new words.

Reading not only allows us to accumulate words, facts, and theories; it expands our consciousness by creating new brain synapses (connections between one neuron and another) and circuits that are honed to generate language. Reading facilitates in a profound way our worldview, allowing us to do more, move in new directions, and live an enriched life.

But what happens to someone who is never given the opportunity to read? It is widely accepted that the opportunities associated with education are huge, and that people deprived of this opportunity are blocked from obtaining mentally stimulating jobs, forced into low-paying manual jobs that are tedious and potentially deleterious to our health. Non-readers make far less money, and 40 percent of our prisons are filled with people who are dyslexic. And not reading is a risk factor for Alzheimer's disease. A neurologist from Belo Horizonte Brazil, Elisa Resende, has shown that in this region, people with less than four years of education have smaller hippocampi. The hippocampi are the structures in the temporal lobes where Alzheimer's disease often begins and where memory is localized. Her work suggests that having a smaller memory system (a memory system blunted by low education and the inability to read) is a risk factor that makes these non-readers vulnerable to Alzheimer's disease.

Jerry Weinstein was not a reader, although he was always excellent in math and other aspects of learning. His Alzheimer's disease began in the reading part of the brain, which manifested with the inability to pull up the word "crouton." When Jerry attended grade school, dyslexia was rarely diagnosed, but one has to wonder whether his disinterest in reading, or possibly even dyslexia, played a role in his presentation of Alzheimer's disease.

While dyslexia or decreased reading by itself are not clearly risks for Alzheimer's disease, neurologists Marilu Gorno Tempini and Zac Miller at UCSF have shown that when non-readers like Jerry get Alzheimer's disease, they are more likely to exhibit early abnormalities in naming, reading, and spelling before memory issues emerge. Diminished reading, even when a person has otherwise normal learning and a high-level occupation, predisposes the person to a type of Alzheimer's disease where the illness begins in the left hemisphere in a region involved with reading and naming. The memory region, the hippocampus, is affected later.

Zac Miller is also showing that other types of learning abnormalities influence the location of Alzheimer's disease. Difficulty with mathematics and spatial navigation in early life is associated with a different type of the disease, one in which the first symptoms are deficits in the visual interpretation of the world. The person is unable to see objects in front of them. Even though their eyes work perfectly, the signals from the eyes to the brain become dysfunctional, and eventually, these patients become, for all intents and purposes, blind. Called posterior cortical atrophy, this version of Alzheimer's disease starts in the most posterior parts of the cortex, posterior parietal, temporal, and even occipital cortex. And, as is true with logopenic aphasia as well, episodic and working memory are initially spared. Furthermore, many patients with posterior cortical atrophy show early-life learning deficiencies.

Many scientists believe that if we had better remedial programs for learning abnormalities when they appeared in childhood, we might stave off the onset of Alzheimer's disease for years in those vulnerable individuals. It is already known that early interventions in cases of learning differences greatly remediate these problems. How a society approaches its most vulnerable learners can influence the appearance of disease later in life. Respect for humans is not only humane, it is cost effective. Intervening early to educate young people is far less costly than treating dementia later in life.

Finally, as Cindy notes, as the disease progresses, Jerry has many symptoms beyond just language, and she ponders whether her father can truly love her even if he has no words to describe the love and has lost the memories of their collective experiences. She realizes how important his love is to her in order to validate her own meaning, existence. She notes, "If someone remembers having loved you, is that the same as them loving you?" Later she goes on, "I say he loved me, but really what I mean is that I think, on some level, he remembered that I was someone he had loved. Even if he didn't know exactly who I was, he knew I was someone who had mattered to him once upon a time."

Her comment is profound, and many caregivers think about similar ideas, sometimes in an agonizing fashion. Another question that the reader might ask is, "Does Cindy's love for her father *before* Alzheimer's disease help him cope with *his* Alzheimer's disease?" Of course, there is no absolute answer, but it won't surprise the reader to know that I have my own opinion that is anatomical, phenomenological, and strongly rooted in behavioral neurology principles.

Based on experience, it is evident that Jerry loves Cindy. She feels it in his face, in his body language, and in his apparent comfort in being with her. This is fairly typical with Alzheimer's disease. Certainly in the early stages of Alzheimer's disease, people usually remain gentle, caring, and empathic, and that is because the circuits of empathy are spared. This is not true in frontotemporal dementia, where many of those afflicted become less loving and less empathic. This loss of empathy and love happens because the circuits of empathy are hit first.

While neuroscientists can't yet tell us what the anatomic substrates of love are, it is evident that there are very distinct circuits in the brain that are critical for the expression and experience of love and empathy. What our face and body shows is strongly associated with what we feel. Affective scientists have found that intentionally smiling makes us feel better and holding our face in a frown can increase sadness and anger (your mom was right). If Jerry seemed to love and want to be with Cindy, even though he lacked memory and language, I don't think we should ignore what we see. Further, the circuitry of love is not critically linked to language or memory, and subcortical and right cerebral hemisphere circuits seem to be more central to this process. In fact, it is even possible that the release of left hemisphere cortical circuits might enhance the function of the deep circuits involved with a father's love for his daughter.

So did Jerry's emotion tell us that he still loved Cindy? I think that it did. I believe that Jerry's love for Cindy remained despite his cognitive deterioration. This part of Jerry's humanity was untouched by this terrible disease. I also believe that Cindy's love for her father stimulated Jerry's circuits in a way that maintained his emotional well-being. Her love was sustaining and meaningful and exemplified what we caregivers can do for our friends and relatives when they become ill.

· 3 ·

Space

Lost in Space

When I got to Berkeley in August of 1982, I found home. The feeling of being in the right place was profound and steadying. Breathing came easier. The coffee stronger. The sky bluer. The library better. At last, I was doing exactly what I had wanted to get back to doing since that summer of 1977 at Phillips Academy Andover when I read twelve books in six weeks. For three blissful years, from 1982 to 1985, I was happier than I'd ever been in my life. All I did was read books and talk about them nonstop. I relished being among people who cared as much as me about novels, narrators, and Vladimir Nabokov.

But my parents, especially my father, weren't happy. My mom was settling into their new place in Florida, and Dad was selling the business he had run with Uncle Bernie, his brother-in-law, for over thirty years. The house in Verona, New Jersey, where my family lived for my entire life, had been sold, and while Dad and Bernie were closing up Apex Electrical Supply Company, the business that brought them monetary success and happiness, more often than not, Dad moved into a friend's garden apartment. The place was packed to the gills with someone else's clothes and furniture, and when Jim and I visited Dad that first year of graduate school, there was barely room to move around. I mostly remember the clunky chairs covered with plastic, and the sadness of seeing Dad living in an old apartment, that kind really old people live in, amidst someone else's stuff. Mind you, the house in Verona where I grew up wouldn't have made it into the pages of *Architectural Digest*, but compared to Dad's new digs, it was paradise. Ironically, the air in that inappropriately named "garden apartment" lacked oxygen. The 1950s heater seemed to have a life of its own, and its baseline temperature hovered around a stultifying 80 degrees.

Dad seemed unhappy, although he didn't say as much. Jim remembers me telling him that Dad was acting differently on that visit, though exactly what seemed off I can't recall. My dim recollection is that it was related to Dad's mood, which I probably chalked up to all of the big changes occurring in Dad's life and the shitbox he was living in. Bruce believes that changes in mood are not reactions to the disease. They are the disease itself. In other words, depression isn't some external response to dementia, but constitutes an aspect of it.

Dad pretended to be okay with the garden apartment and resigned to occupying a domestic space different than the one he had spent much of his adult life in. After all, it was temporary. I can only imagine how unanchored he must have felt with the double whammy of simultaneously selling the house and the business. He was retiring from Apex Electrical Supply, an enterprise that he had put his heart and soul into in order to give me, Mom, my sister, and brother everything we could possibly want—especially a limitless amount of love. He poured his all into that business and then gave it all to us. Linda went to Princeton (God, they were so proud of her—she was in one of the first classes that accepted women) and then George Washington Law School; Lyle went to Wesleyan and then the

University of Colorado Boulder Law School, proudly paying for most of this by himself, but still knew there was financial support waiting in the wings, should he need it; and then me. Brandeis undergraduate; Berkeley for graduate school.

The bottom line, the sad paradox that this chapter will describe, is that just as I found my space in Berkeley, Dad lost his. It was a matter of time until he quite literally started getting lost. And when that happened, I got lost. Where was home? I didn't want to leave Berkeley but staying was brutal on the conscience and has been for a very long time.

I'm writing these words about Berkeley in Berkeley, having left southern California for a year to study neurology and, truth be told, to revisit my decision to remain here all those years ago. My therapist has encouraged me to forgive myself for the decisions I made in my twenties. This is not easy. She has suggested that I psychically reposition myself away from guilt and work toward the less judgmental idea of regret. Imagine the salt and pepper shakers on the table except instead of an S and a P, there is a G and an R. One for guilt, the other for regret. I have been refilling the guilt one for what feels like forever. Regret has remained untouched. Anyway, she thinks my psychic spice rack needs some readjusting. I suppose that's one way to understand this book.

In this chapter, though, I want to describe what it looked like when my dad was losing his way. Two very specific memories sear my mind: the first takes place in one of the casual restaurants, like a diner, in the Frontier Hotel in Las Vegas, and the second on the Poinciana golf course in Lake Worth, Florida. Looking back at my reaction to my father's spatial disorientation makes me wonder what I was thinking. Scratch that, I know what I was thinking. It was a desperate attempt to respond to his dislocation by locating myself as deeply (and I thought safely) in my intellectual, novel-loving, aesthetically pleasing space. Funnily enough, feeling the pain would have been the smarter approach to take. And then I try to remind myself that maybe this was the best I could do.

Before getting to Las Vegas, I should say that my father had a beautifully attuned sense of direction. I remember when he was in his forties, he would drive me, hugging the road and always and forever emotionally hugging me, to my piano lesson once a week in his little yellow five-speed, stick-shift hatchback Datsun that got over thirty miles to the gallon. My dad listened to Jimmy Carter when he said to conserve energy. Years later, my driving-loving father could no longer drive both because he didn't know how to anymore, and he probably would have killed someone if we had let him behind the wheel. If you couldn't read the letters making up the word S-T-O-P, chances are you should not be in the driver's seat ready to G-O. We told him the car was broken and couldn't be repaired. And he believed it. Even without the car, whose odometer told the tale of short errands becoming endless travails and drives to neighbors morphing into trips to strangers, he was lost in space. I inherited the last car he drove and was convinced that when the odometer read 90,000 miles, my father would be dead. It seemed like the right ending. The way a novel would end. Sadly, Dad outlived the car.

•   •

The Las Vegas memory is this. After all these years, it remains so close to the surface of my mind that I have to narrate it in the present tense. My mother, father (fifty-eight years old), and I are sitting at a booth in a restaurant having breakfast. I am across from them. We are at one of those coffee shop kinds of places that most casinos have. Interestingly, we were staying at the Frontier Hotel. I say interesting because one of the items on my orals list was Frederick Jackson Turner's "The Significance of the Frontier in American History" (1893), a historical work whose significance to this chapter will become clear. The restaurant is quiet, strangely so because everything in Las Vegas blares, with the exception of those weird baccarat rooms, hidden in the back of the casino, that exude the silence of the extraordinarily wealthy for whom losing or winning millions at a time makes no difference. Milling about the main area of the casino, one hears the slot machines shriek, the gamblers guffaw or sigh mightily, and the volume of the music is turned up so high that you can't hear what the person next to you is saying. I recall walking through the casino with Dad and hearing "New York, New York," a song we both liked but could barely enjoy because Frank Sinatra's voice seemed strangely aggressive in its loudness. The whole experience is the equivalent of a sonic assault, which leads me to think that maybe the quiet I am remembering is made up because when what I am about to describe happened, time stopped and sound did, too.

My father's pancakes arrive, and the little maple syrup cups—you know the kind that you used to get at Howard Johnson's in the containers that you played with by stacking them one on top of the other until the pancakes or waffles came—are in front of him. Cups, containers, packets. The thingies that I am trying to describe are so unnatural and bogus, like the syrup in them, that they're not even called any one thing. You need a bunch of words just to get close to the object that the words can't even name. Anyway, at this point in his illness, we could still pretend that Dad could do things for himself because sometimes he could. Sometimes he did know how to dress himself even if his clothes needed to be laid out on the bed so he wouldn't try to put on two pairs of pants. Sometimes he could get the food on the fork and bring it to his mouth, and we didn't need to pretend that it was okay to treat all foods like finger food. But one never knew what was around the bend. One never knew what he wouldn't know and when he

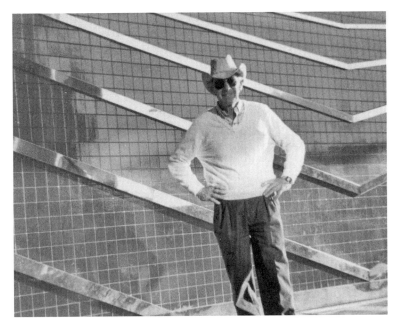

Jerry in Las Vegas, 1986

wouldn't know it (and when he would remember it again only
to forget it again once and for all).

Well, what was around the bend on this Thanksgiving break
was not that he no longer knew how to put film in the camera. Nor was it that he no longer walked, but rather shuffled.
No, it was the maple syrup. The waitress brought our food, and
my mom and I started eating our breakfast until we noticed
that Dad wasn't doing much of anything with his pancakes. I
asked Dad if he wanted maple syrup on his pancakes, and he
said yes, and I pointed out to him where the packets were. The
idea being that rather than getting it for him, opening it, and
pouring it on the pancakes (perhaps this task or tasks were still
something he knew how to do), he could do this for himself
and have the sense of accomplishment that came with one less
thing needing to be done for him. He nodded his head and

picked up the packet, as if understanding, and I approvingly nodded back. God knows how many times my mom had been through a version of this. She was quietly trying to enjoy her meal. Besides this was a "vacation" for her, and I was there and could help to relieve her of this one small bit of awfulness.

But I couldn't. With maple syrup packet in hand, Dad made the correct motion to pour it over his pancakes. He waited patiently, waiting for the syrup to come out, like when the ketchup takes a while to make it to the French fries. He shook the packet thinking perhaps, and I'm obviously guessing here, that it had coagulated and that's why it wasn't coming out. But it wasn't coming out because he hadn't opened it. He held the packet over the pancakes waiting for the syrup to emerge, but the syrup was locked up in its stupid plastic thingama-bob. It was like a Marcel Marceau pantomime skit. Everything was silent, and he was acting out a sketch of a person pouring maple syrup on his pancakes. But of course, he wasn't perform-ing, or rather, he was. He was performing knowing what to do with that packet of syrup until he couldn't perform any longer. What came out of the packet was not the syrup, but the fact that he had no idea what he was doing. In other words, what emerged was nothing or, more precisely, the coagulated noth-ingness that was my father's mind (obviously, another guess).

Like Huck Finn, who escapes from the confines of Widow Douglas's religion and discipline, I wanted to light out for a ter-ritory and leave my suffering behind. Out of the Frontier cof-fee shop to somewhere else, even Caesar's Palace or God forbid, Circus, Circus, but I couldn't physically do that. And I couldn't burst into tears. My father didn't seem to realize there was a problem, so I didn't want to upset him by bawling my eyes out, and my mother couldn't bear to see my pain. I couldn't leave and I couldn't stay. Thus, I did what any self-respecting aca-demic would do and ran and hid in my intellect. The moment,

I apprehended, had the quality of a surrealist painting. This observation struck me, and still does, as both true and completely irrelevant. The insight also functioned strategically. It allowed me simultaneously to remain in place and be somewhere else—a nice description of reading. You're there but not. This was my steady state from the time I learned my father had Alzheimer's disease. I was in Berkeley, but I wasn't. I was reading *The Scarlet Letter* and thinking Dad.

In that moment when confronted by my father's illness in the shape of a piece of unopened plastic that contained a plastic-like substance that some company called "syrup," I turned away or turned inward. This is what Alzheimer's looked like in the Frontier Hotel, but I made it look like something else in order to make it bearable. To look at my father's disease directly would have been like looking at the sun during an eclipse. I would have gone blind or at least that's what I thought at the time. I didn't or couldn't or wouldn't look straight at it, but rather positioned myself at an angle whose maintenance, in that moment and over many years, required all of my intellectual and emotional strength to sustain in order I would have no energy left to feel.

I approached this moment as if it were something to be analyzed. Thus, like René Magritte's picture of a pipe with the words, "Ceci n'est pas une pipe," the image of my father would have been accompanied by a Luigi Pirandello–inspired dramatic title, such as *Six Pancakes in Search of Some Syrup* or *Naked Brunch*, a riff on William Burroughs's *Naked Lunch*. The point being that nothing in reality could prepare a daughter for seeing her father fail to know that pouring syrup on pancakes requires that he open the piece of plastic so the syrup will come out. I made a picture of my Alzheimer's-inflicted dad with the Magritte-inspired caption, "Ceci n'est pas Alzheimer's." Only art could help me survive this onslaught of reality.

The frontier I lit out for was my imagination or, more precisely, the imaginations of others I was studying. Which brings me back to 1893 and Turner's frontier thesis, which he presented to the American Historical Association at its Chicago meeting. The argument turns on the importance of territorial expansion to the making of American identity and the belief that Americans are exceptional. The frontier inspires Americans to do great things and provides unlimited opportunities for the accomplishment of great deeds. Never mind that such heroic acts involved decimating native people or animal populations. Turner worries that with the closing of the frontier, the can-do American spirit will shrivel up, and the antidote to this entails the conquest of new lands. Hawaii. The Philippines. Iraq.

My favorite part of Turner's thesis has to do with his account of how the frontier functioned as a "safety valve" for Americans. The idea, both creative and utterly wrongheaded (hence, my favorite), being that when urban centers became intolerably overcrowded, and the myth of America as a classless society became impossible to sustain (sometimes the work ethic just means more work and not an opportunity to make a better life), a person could always go west. The West symbolized possibility, an opening to perpetual transformation, a geography—a nation or a person—waiting to come into being. Of course, it already had existed well before Turner claimed it hadn't, and many Native Americans lived there, but that was beside his point.

I went to Berkeley for these things, too, but rather than thinking in terms of a "safety valve," I had in mind an episode from the Jerry Seinfeld show, where George gleefully announces that his parents will be moving to Florida, creating a twelve-hundred-mile buffer zone between them and him. Mine would be significantly bigger. A three thousand-mile buffer zone, a safety valve, as it were, between me and my parents seemed like just the thing as I was embarking on what I most wanted to do with my life (read). Until my father started losing his mind and I started losing mine. The safety valve wasn't so safe, after all. My frontier, like Turner's, was already occupied, in my case by the ghosts of my father's dying memory. And so, I found another frontier, filled with books, where I could jam my mind with knowledge and novels and words to counteract the daily loss of just those things that my dad was experiencing. If Dad's mind was like a colander that couldn't retain anything or like a tire that kept leaking air, my mind was busily trying to plug the holes (where were they?) by reading books. How stupid is that? It made perfect sense at the time. It was a race to keep emptiness at a distance.

The second memory, the one I remember despite not having been there, takes place on a golf course in Florida. Whenever my father would talk about his ideal retirement years, he would conjure up his days as a series of perpetual rounds of golf. He looked down on the players who rode around in golf carts. He preferred to walk the eighteen holes. In addition to enjoying the chitchat with the caddies who walked the course and shlepped the clubs (my poor brother was often among them), I think this had a lot to do, ironically, with his desire to do everything he could to stay healthy. For example, after reading a particularly horrific article about the use of antibiotics in cattle, he swore off red meat. He jogged three miles a day for decades and took lots of vitamins. And man was he healthy—physically, that is. That would come back to bite him in the ass when it took his body over a decade to get to that empty place where his mind had gotten to so many years before.

My father played golf when he wasn't working: on the weekends in New Jersey, on vacation in Las Vegas, in Florida. Looking back, we had a glimpse, albeit a humorous one, of the hazards of organizing one's vacations, let alone one's life, around Dad's penchant for golf. The scene is Jekyll Island in Georgia, a touristic cul-de-sac (sinkhole or sewer might be more accurate), popular among deluded suburbanites in the 1970s. Jekyll Island, by the way, has no connection whatsoever to Robert Louis Stevenson's 1886 *Strange Case of Dr. Jekyll and Mr. Hyde*. That said, the story of a person having two identities resonates. In the Stevenson classic, Dr. Jekyll is an upstanding, cerebral medic, happy to be part of his community. Mr. Hyde the hedonistic, violent-lusting other, happy to inflict pain on others. When the identities refuse to remain in their compartments, things fall apart. Hence, the personal resonance, which thankfully was less about content (among my many flaws, a lust for violence is not one of them) and more about structure: daughter goes here, literary critic goes there. Also, Jekyll Island advertised itself as a vacation paradise, which it was not.

I remember having very little to do during that vacation because it rained like crazy, making it impossible to swim in the pool or play tennis or shuffleboard. Instead, I made my way through Charles Dickens's *Great Expectations*, which my mother told me I had to finish before I could read the book I really wanted to read—Erich Segal's *Love Story*. I liked Dickens well enough, but a highlight of the vacation (to give you a sense of the awfulness of this vacation from the perspective of a ten-year-old) was taking a break from Pip's adventures in England and watching Lew Alcindor of the Milwaukee Bucks on the television (Alcindor had yet to become Kareem Abdul-Jabbar or a Los Angeles Laker). During what seemed like a hurricane of a rainstorm outside, I also recall a car ride to a restaurant that catered to tourists. The radio in the background blared Gladys Knight and the Pips's "Rainy Night in Georgia" (or was it "Midnight Train to Georgia"?). By the way, I have no doubt that I am here making synchronic or simultaneous a couple of moments that happened sequentially. I cannot resist allowing for the possibility that Pip's name might hopscotch from Dickens to Gladys Knight and of course there's Herman Melville's "Pip," the character in *Moby-Dick* who jumps into the ocean while chasing a whale and goes mad.

In any case, not only could my dad not play much golf on Jekyll Island during that vacation of the squall, but also the family could barely breathe. We slept, or tried to, with our faces scrunched up into the pillows so as to take in a minimum amount of air. Turns out, a toxic odor was Jekyll Island's Mr. Hyde. The hotel where we stayed, which the brochures somehow failed to mention, was nestled close to a chemical factory that belched out sulfuric-smelling winds. Imagine, if you will, all of the eggs in the egg section of Costco—say the one in Boca Raton—having been hardboiled, left unrefrigerated to marinate in the profound humidity of south Florida, and, as a result, exuding the stench of thousands of rotten eggs. This image gives you some idea of the breadth, the inescapability, the ghastly redolence of our Jekyll Island holiday.

Next to Georgia is Florida, and in Florida is Lake Worth (worth what?), and in Lake Worth is the golf course, the site of the second memory that bookends this chapter. Poinciana was the name of the retirement village my parents lived in, and it had a golf course where my father loved to play with his friends until he couldn't remember how to play and didn't have any friends left. Not because he didn't know them at that point in his illness, but *they* couldn't bear to know *him*. This is called stigma. People fear others who are ill, as if that illness might be contagious. For those people and their loved ones, being stigmatized is painful. Not as painful as the illness itself, but still.

Dad had a lot of friends when he could play and remember where he was, but people can only withstand witnessing so much dissolution and suffering before they jump ship. Invitations to play golf, to play cards, to go out to dinner as a couple, started drying up. My mother couldn't understand why. She finally found out one day when she innocently asked one of Dad's golf partners why he hadn't been playing much lately. He replied that he had been playing, and then explained the reason for my father being excluded. Bottom line: the men couldn't take it anymore.

Apparently, there had been difficulties for a while (my mother didn't go into details, perhaps because my dad's friend didn't, perhaps because she wanted to spare me), but the straw that broke the camel's back for the group of men with whom my dad had been playing golf for decades was the following. He had the golf club in hand ready to swing for the fences, except he was literally swinging for and at the fences. In other words, he was aiming away from the putting green, positioning himself in the exact wrong direction. One of the men in the group gently turned my father's body around, correcting the error, helping my dad to finish the round, the last round he would play.

That's it. That's the memory, which combines kindness and cruelty in a way that I have never been able to put my finger on. Maybe because everyone in the memory does the best they can, but that does nothing to change the awful result. The kindness lies in the act of an older man gently (I remember that was the word my mother used) putting his hands around my father's waist (okay, I'm inventing here) and wordlessly turning him around so he could take the swing. The man would do this one kind thing and never more (no relation to "Nevermore" in Edgar Allan Poe's "The Raven") put himself in a situation where he would have to do it again. When my mother told me about this over the phone, I cursed up a blue streak and then signed up to take golf lessons at a driving range not

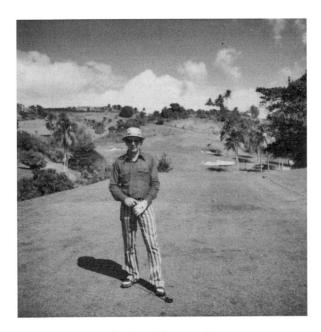

Jerry playing golf (year unknown)

far from the Berkeley campus. I have slightly more sympathy
for Dad's golf partners now than at the time. I think they were
frightened, that somehow Dad's illness was catching. Plus they
were men in their sixties, born in the twenties, and not your
typical caregiving population. If they wouldn't play golf with
Dad because his illness was interfering with their good time,
I would pick up the slack. Somehow. I would do that from the
other side of the country, while teaching a composition class
and writing my dissertation. And somehow learning to play
golf three thousand miles away from my father translated into
playing golf with my father.

Reality was clearly beside the point. As a teenager, I had tried
to learn how to play golf once before. After all, it was so important to my father that I thought if I could learn how to play, it

would make him happy and give us more stuff to do together. Dad decided to teach me. A mistake on the order of him teaching me how to drive a stick shift, which, unlike golf, I did eventually master. To cut to the chase, the two of us became so frustrated with my ineptitude that my companionship on the golf course devolved into me throwing the golf ball from one part of the green to the next while Dad laughingly showed off his beautiful swing to a humbled but delighted daughter.

Golf ran in my father's DNA. Alzheimer's probably did too. After my father's diagnosis, we had a different understanding of the mishmash of stuff we discovered in my nana and pop's (our names for my father's mother and father) garage. When we went through their belongings to move them from New Jersey to Florida and found hidden wads of cash in suitcases that hadn't been opened for thirty years or bottles of ketchup that had been bought years before and never used and stored with the cash in the suitcases, we attributed this kooky mess to my pop's love of gambling and fear of my nana knowing about his extracurricular gambling hobby. He was hiding the cash acquired from bets made on the horses at the racetrack. The ketchup was something different, but we didn't know exactly what to call it. We used a verbal placeholder and called it odd. Like my dad's worsening handwriting, the chaotic juxtaposition of things in my pop's suitcases was probably a symptom.

Even when the disease presented itself, which it uncannily did in the form of a funny story that made no sense, with golf making a surprise appearance, we still didn't know what to call it. Here's the background. My nana fell outside of her apartment building in New Jersey and broke her hip. My pop was obviously affected by her injury because for a while he didn't go to work so that he could take care of her. In his later years, he worked as a driver in my father's business, and God knows how many packages never made it to their destination or how much extra gas had to be bought because he got lost. Anyway, Nana fell into a really big pothole, which the landlord knew about but hadn't fixed despite our many attempts to get him to do the right thing. Dad hired a lawyer, who went after the morally deficient landlord. We had a good case. Clearly the victims, both in their seventies, my injured (and ornery) nana and my sweet pop, with his loving smile and quirky sense of humor, only had to say what happened, the pain she experienced from the fall, and the things he could no longer enjoy because of her injury. Picturing my pop now, I'm seeing Rip Van Winkle, with my nana, I'm afraid, playing the shrewish Dame Van Winkle. I should add that in her later years, she mellowed out, with the help of the vodka we would sneak into the nursing home.

At the hearing, my nana knew what to say, plus her broken hip spoke for itself. The lawyer had coached my pop several times, drilling him on what he should and shouldn't say and what he might be asked about. For good measure, my father also went over the narrative of events, but now I think maybe it wasn't for good measure, but rather it was because my dad didn't have confidence that his father could keep the story straight; in other words, that Pop might not remember what happened. And he couldn't. When my father came home from the deposition that night, I was first at the door. I took one look at him and quickly poured him a drink. I hadn't seen him that angry since my brother pulled the car out of the garage but forgot to open the garage door first. My mom, Dad, and I sat at the kitchen table, and Dad recounted what happened.

Everything went according to the script, at first. Pop described bringing the pothole to the landlord's attention, followed by his account of Nana's fall and then not being able to work. And then Pop was asked a simple follow-up question.

"What are you unable to do after your wife's fall that you were able to do prior to the fall?"

My pop correctly said he could not work anymore.

"What else?" said our lawyer.

"Play golf," replied Pop.

At this moment in the retelling, I thought my father might have a heart attack, and so I took out the bottle of vodka and poured him another shot. My father continued.

The lawyer then asked, "How often did you play golf?"

Pop replied, "Never."

My dad couldn't help but laugh—and cry a little—as he recounted the exchange that resulted in my nana and pop receiving a minimal settlement that did little to improve their quality of life in their retirement years. It goes without saying that Nana and Pop were quite pleased with their performance at the deposition.

I had this story in my mind about my pop when I took my first golf lesson in Berkeley. I also had in mind the time when I threw the golf ball with my dad laughing at me and me at myself. Jekyll Island was in there somewhere. Also in my mind was Robert Pirsig's *Zen and the Art of Motorcycle Maintenance* because it struck me that his advice about motorcycle maintenance and self-care might apply to my feelings about golf and to me. In Pirsig's company, I thought I was prepared to overcome whatever physical and mental obstacles had previously prevented me from being able to hit a tiny ball that wasn't moving. I tried to surrender my ego to the power of the ball. I tried to let thoughts float in and out of my mind without attaching feelings to them. I tried to have no expectations, no fear of failure. I sucked at that. I did just what Pirsig says you're not supposed to do. The ball quickly became my enemy, like Odysseus and the Cyclops, and it was only a hop, skip, and a jump (and several failed swings) before I became my enemy. My thoughts screeched, and I couldn't let them be and then be gone. I did everything wrong. I adopted an ironic position toward the ball: how come I can hit a tennis ball going fast and I can't hit you, who is just sitting there mocking me in your immobility? I tried anger: I'm going to hit this fucking ball and when I do, I'm never coming back to this driving range. I despaired: I can't hit the ball and I'm never going to be able to leave the driving range. I whiffed, sweated, muttered, and left the range a defeated woman.

Why on earth I thought my father's illness would be the thing that would finally allow me to connect golf club with golf ball (for Chrissakes, I wasn't even very good at miniature golf) is beyond comprehension. And why I thought Pirsig would help, too, strikes me now as utterly irrational. Signing up for that lesson, thinking that my whole history with golf would somehow right itself through sheer force of literary will and hermeneutic expertise, was clearly an emotional Hail Mary pass. Not only were my tears getting in the way of seeing the actual ball, but the fact remained that, like years before, I still couldn't get the hang of holding the damned golf club. That piece of wood or iron has to be one of the most counter-intuitive pieces of equipment used for play ever invented by a human being. I can only chalk up my deeply flawed belief that I would magically be able to hold the club and hit the ball to my inhabiting the world of fiction, where the protagonist, like Hercules, must suffer all sorts of setbacks only to be rewarded at the end of the story with success. In other words, golf was no longer golf. It was overdetermined—by Jekyll Island, by my previous attempt to play, by my pop's testimony—so when I showed up at that lesson in Berkeley, golf had come to symbolize not only my relationship with my father but also a way to overcome his illness. Connecting club to ball was connecting me to him. If I couldn't do it, he was lost. If I could, he wasn't. All the maintenance in the world wasn't going to help.

On another level, though, I knew better. The books I loved

best didn't end well. Sure, Ishmael makes it, but no one else does. Atop Moby Dick, Ahab dies strangled to death by harpoon lines. Vladimir Nabokov's Humbert Humbert dies and so does Lolita, emotionally shattered by years of having been sexually assaulted. Benjy, the castrated, thirty-three-year-old mentally handicapped character who cries away his days missing his sister and his testicles, in William Faulkner's *The Sound and the Fury*, survives, but his brother Quentin commits suicide and his father and uncle die alcoholics.

I bring up Faulkner's 1929 novel (the year my mother was born, two years after my father) for two reasons: the first being that I love it for its narrative experimentation and its powerful diagnosis of slavery as the cause of the South's downfall; and the second being that golf makes an appearance. In fact, the novel opens with a scene on a golf course, where there are caddies and balls. In the Compson family of Faulkner's Yoknapatawpha County, "caddy" means only one thing, and it isn't the person carrying the golf clubs. Caddy is the name of Benjy's sister, the sister with whom all of the brothers are in love. She has escaped the Compson family, revealing its inability to process her loss and carry on. And "balls" means only one thing. Benjy's missing ones. When Benjy hears someone calling out "caddy," he cries because that word refers to an absence. When he looks at his body in the mirror, he weeps for what has been lost. When I teach *The Sound and the Fury*, I must be careful not to cry in front of my students lest I have to explain to them how golf, for me, has come to signify the loss of my father. How the character of Benjy contains both my sadness (my dad is gone) and my projection of my father's sadness (his experience of having lost so much).

For better or worse, these were the stories that drew me in. Only in a novel—and one that I probably didn't like—could a girl who couldn't hit a golf ball to save her life suddenly be able to hit one because she so loved her father, who had been diagnosed with Alzheimer's disease and loved golf, that that love transcended the fact that she and golf simply didn't get along. Never had. Never would. Or rather, they only got along in stories, brought to life by the conjunction of my imagination and others', that, when strung together, made for a narrative with golf appearing, once in a while, in comic and tragic relief.

Two Kinds of Space

We often take our parents for granted, demanding their nurturance while treating their talents as foibles or idiosyncrasies that irritate or embarrass us. Yet, when faced with the threat or reality of a parent's loss, this perspective often changes, and we quickly redefine our opinions in a more positive light. "Don't it always seem to go that you don't know what you got till it's gone," sings the great Joni Mitchell. My father played piano by ear—hear it once, and it was there for good. How many fathers can do that, and where did that skill come from in the brain? I never pondered those questions during his life, always figuring that the piano playing was just what we got with Dad. It was part of what Cindy would call his "space." Sadly, rarely did Dad's playing give me joy. At best it was a background sound in our house, sometimes an annoying one.

This process of diminishing valuation with each response is called habituation. Get the same stimulus enough times, and the response to it progressively diminishes. Once-pleasant stimuli become unpleasant with steady repetition. This happens with food, music, sex, drugs, you name it, and scientists understand this process of habituation down to the single synapse. Admittedly, my inability to appreciate my father's piano playing was more complicated than simple habituation. I was a little envious and competitive with Dad, and it was harder for me to root for him than it should have been. After one listen, he could spontaneously play and sing almost any song ranging from Lerner and Loewe's whole musical *My Fair Lady* to Whitney Houston's "Didn't We Almost Have It All." Whitney Houston was his all-time favorite. Dad really wanted us to "have it all," and he had a remarkable passion for living. I wish I could hear him play and sing Whitney Houston one more time, but my dad has been gone for fifteen years, and my ninety-four-year-old mother for the first time is sick. So, the "all" that we had together as a family is vanishing. Soon all that will remain for me will be memories—many of them twisted and distorted with the passage of time. And eventually those will also go. Cindy's father clearly wanted her to "have it all," and she wanted this for him. With Alzheimer's disease, Jerry lost everything. That's what happens with Alzheimer's disease.

A loving father and parent, Jerry had many talents prior to getting sick. He was an excellent driver with an uncanny ability to navigate, and he was also an accomplished golfer and gambler. Skills like these frame our lives, and most of us seek out situations where our skills can be practiced and honed. Jerry spent his weekends and vacations focused upon the hobbies that he enjoyed, visiting golf courses in New Jersey and Florida and gambling in Las Vegas. If Jerry had worn an actigraph, a monitor that tracked his every movement, it would capture his pathways to the places that he loved—a quantitative measure of the essence of Jerry—his "space." Jerry's deterioration in golf and in gambling was particularly cruel, as these games were critically important to his pride about who he was. William James called these aspects of our mind—the part that is at the core of who we are—the "me self." For James, the "me self" represented our constellation of preferences, self-constructs, religious beliefs, political affiliations, taste in colors, and dress—all of our unique identifiers. Jerry's love for golf and gambling were not activities that Cindy enjoyed. Despite her love for her father, her "me self" contained different hobbies, beliefs, and skill sets.

It is no surprise that passion and skill go together. If we enjoy an activity, we are more likely to do it frequently and, in turn, we become progressively more accomplished at performing that activity. The author Malcolm Gladwell has noted that we need to practice an activity ten thousand times before true mastery of that skill occurs. With Cindy's antipathy to golf, she never came close to the ten thousand times. In general, it's those things that we love that we are inclined to practice enough to do in an exceptional way.

Learning a skill activates multiple brain regions, including the motor portions of the cortex that help carry out voluntary commands, and the basal ganglia and the cerebellum, regions where the movements are unconsciously organized. For example, a golf swing has a conscious component commanded by the cortex, but to swing perfectly, those unconscious deep circuits in the basal ganglia and cerebellum need to be activated. Sports psychologists understand this process and work with athletes to drive skills deep in the brain with repetitive practice. The more we practice, the more easily we access these unconscious circuits.

Once we excel at something, others are more likely to recognize and reward us with praise and admiration. This praise is reinforcing, but for the things that we do with real passion, like my father's piano-playing or Jerry's golfing, the activity itself is its own reward. Why Cindy preferred reading, while her father enjoyed golf and gambling, comes down simply to brain wiring, wiring that is present very early in life, even in utero, before we are born. Children are remarkably different in what they pursue and accomplish, and the term "neurodiversity" has been coined to capture this heterogeneity in human abilities and interests. A wonderful expression, neurodiversity is by its very definition tolerant and democratic, acknowledging that we are all different and that we all have our own unique strengths and weaknesses. By five, I was already a voracious reader indifferent to the nuances of machines, while, by contrast, at one year of age my grandson Mason was already trying to figure out how his toys were put together. Now six, he is a master of Legos, putting together ships and airplanes designed for a child who is twelve or older.

Brain wiring in the left hemisphere is important for language, while the right hemisphere, particularly the right posterior temporal-parietal regions, helps us to navigate, draw, gamble, and fix machines. The pursuit of left- or right-hemisphere-localized activities can be introduced, encouraged, and even stimulated by parents when a child is at an early age, but there are also innate brain wiring components to preference. Such preferences usually persist throughout our lifetime. As the study of dementia is showing, sometimes our strengths enhance our weaknesses, while our weaknesses bring out specific strengths. The study of neurodiversity is just beginning.

My work with patients who developed new artistic skills in the setting of dementia sheds light on how brain wiring drives what we do, eventually leading to a nuanced definition of our "me self." The surprising finding is that, in some patients who suffer selective degeneration in their language hemisphere, skills residing in the right hemisphere, in particular, drawing, painting, and sculpting, mysteriously emerge. Jack, a banker with no interest in art suddenly began to paint obsessively. He painted parrots, fish, and sailboats, with striking use of his two favorite colors: purple and yellow. Sadly, these new interests and abilities came in the setting of progressive loss of language along with the loss of knowledge about the meaning of words. At the time that these skills emerged, we learned that Jack's left anterior temporal lobe was degenerating due to what we now call semantic variant primary progressive aphasia. As the left side of the brain shuts down, the right side becomes more active. By contrast, the emergence of obsessive writing, punning, or speaking, left hemisphere activities, can appear with the degeneration of the right anterior temporal lobe.

These surprising findings have led us to believe that a balance between activities in the left versus the right anterior temporal neurons is the driver for preference. These dramatic shifts in interest typically occur in frontotemporal dementia, a degenerative disease that attacks the anterior parts of the brain, including the anterior temporal lobes. By contrast, Alzheimer's disease begins in the hippocampus and the posterior temporal-parietal regions. With Alzheimer's disease, Jerry's illness, the anterior temporal regions that define our preferences seem to be preserved. If we like modern art but dislike art of the Renaissance, this preference persists even late into the illness. Or if we enjoy watching baseball but find football abhorrent, we will continue to watch baseball and walk out of the room whenever football is on the screen.

By contrast, the posterior parietal regions so critical for painting, golf, working with numbers, and naming are preferentially injured with Alzheimer's disease. Therefore, talents accumulated over a lifetime quickly deteriorate. While Jerry's losses in naming, which are localized to the left posterior cortex, were disabling, it was the loss of right posterior cortical functions that truly defined his tragedy. Jerry's "space"—his unique place in the universe—begins to dissipate. The desire to golf, drive a car, and gamble remains, but the skill to perform these activities disappears.

Jerry begins to get lost and no longer knows where to hit his golf balls or where to find them once he has hit them. Jerry is losing spatial skills that were previously sources of great strength. Visuospatial problems are common in Alzheimer's disease and can be placed onto specific anatomical structures in the brain. Determining how spatial memory works, how we navigate a place in the world, brought a Nobel Prize in 2014 to John O'Keefe from England, and May-Britt and Edvard Moser from Norway. Their work was carried out in mice, where they determined what structures help the mouse navigate a maze and elucidated how mice develop a map of their world. Many of the findings from this work focused upon the hippocampus, the small seahorse-shaped neuronal structure in the temporal lobe, where Alzheimer's disease begins. The implications of these findings for human memory and for Alzheimer's disease are undeniable and are described in the final chapter of this book.

The study of spatial memory in rodents was accelerated by psychologist Richard Morris, who became famous for designing a maze that is now extensively used to evaluate how an animal learns to navigate. The Morris Maze is a deep circular pool filled with an opaque liquid into which a rodent, typically a mouse, is placed. The mouse is forced to swim until it can find an invisible platform upon which it is able to stand, allowing it to escape from a tiring swim. Mice hate swimming, so the reward for finding the platform is strong. If the mouse's hippocampus works well, it can quickly learn where the platform sits by rapidly swimming through the maze, avoiding the spaces in the pool that it has already explored. How quickly the mouse learns to find the platform, and how long they remember where it is placed, is determined by how well the hippocampus is working. Mice without hippocampi will never remember where the platform is placed, and when they find the platform it is only by chance, not through a systematic search. This Morris Maze paradigm is highly reminiscent of Alzheimer's disease, where the patient cannot find their car in a parking lot or gets lost driving home. We, like mice, navigate with our hippocampi.

O'Keefe and colleagues demonstrated that there are place cells in the hippocampus that fire as a mouse learns to navigate across an environment and as it develops its own map of the world. Every spot through which the mouse has navigated has place cells that fire each and every time a specific area is passed. When scientists place recording electrodes in the hippocampus during sleep, these same place cells fire when the mouse dreams about moving through the space that it has previously learned. Sleeping and rehearsing the map help a mouse to remember, and the same cells that fired in the dream fire every time the mouse is in a specific place in the maze. What a remarkable system for reinforcing and shaping memory. The mouse maps pathways explored while awake and then rehearses them again during sleep. In mice, both the left and right sides of the hippocampus participate equally in navigation, but in humans, the right side appears to be more important for remembering space, while the left side is specialized for learning new words and for pulling them out of the left hemisphere language regions. Alzheimer's disease hits both regions simultaneously, explaining why Jerry's memory for words and places is disappearing.

Pals from a lifetime of golfing together abandon Jerry the moment that he turns the wrong direction to drive a golf ball. Alzheimer's disease is often a litmus test for our humanity, a test that Jerry's friends in his golfing fraternity badly failed, scoring an F in empathy, friendship, helping, courage, and inner strength. If Jerry is going to recapture the fun that he had golfing or gambling, Cindy is the only hope. Yet, the very idea of golf or gambling is alien to her. Cindy's "space" is quite different from Jerry's. Worse, for her, the casinos and golf courses, where these activities need to happen, smell of decay. Las Vegas, Atlantic City, and the golf courses of New Jersey, glittery places of hope and play for new American immigrants in the 1930s, '40s, and '50s, seem old and stale to the children of these immigrants. These children, like Cindy, need new dreams and playgrounds, not places where their parents and grandparents are dying. Spaces of hope for one generation become reminders of the inevitability of death for another.

Dementia, with its relentless erasing of what we do well and not so well, is often a reckoning for a patient's loved ones. This is who my dad was, this is what I knew about our relationship, and this is me in comparison. Alzheimer's disease challenges concepts around our own "space" and chips away at our confidence. No longer is our parent a steady rock that supports our life, a support that consciously and unconsciously buoys us up. Self-reflections, and reflections about who our loved one is and is becoming, emerge like scenes in a sad novel. In this book, every month, the loved one is different. It happens fast, and the accounting must be repeated over and over again. Alzheimer's disease, and really any serious chronic illness in a person we love, forces us to know that our time is short. We too will pass, maybe in the same sad way. Our "space" will disappear.

It seems insensitive to say that there is something good that happens as Jerry loses his personal space and comfort zone while simultaneously losing his ability to navigate. The pain for Cindy and Jerry is excruciating, almost impossible to measure. It is also a time when loved ones try to understand, reach out, learn, and develop new skills. Jerry's fast friends who abandon him at his first moment of vulnerability are the biggest losers in this story. Their own brain systems for caring, learning about Alzheimer's disease, and deepening their own altruism suffer, and they become forever less, much less. Cindy's act of engagement broadens her vision. She taps an inner strength, a circuitry required for our survival, bringing a new and stronger self for future crises.

· 4 ·

Behavior

Turning Right

Bruce has asked me to write a chapter about behavior. My dad's. I don't want to. There is the difficulty of remembering this aspect of his disease (me Berkeley; him Florida), the pain of doing so, and the sinking feeling that I won't be able to find the right words. I believe that I have managed to come up with a vocabulary to explain my father's loss of his, but I am not confident that my words can fully capture how his early-onset Alzheimer's manifested itself in particular behaviors. Although I don't know if my father did any of the kinds of behaviors Bruce sees in frontotemporal dementia, like crawling on the floor, touching strangers in inappropriate ways, eating packages of sugar because of a sweet tooth, he may have. But I never witnessed anything like that. Those behaviors are more compulsive and brutally physical than the comparatively gentle, but nonetheless traumatic, ones I've already described. Behaviors are embodied in that you see them; language is abstracted in that you hear it. You don't have to be present to hear the logopenic variant of Alzheimer's disease. Its full effects are direct and evident in phone calls.

Of course, you can hear about behaviors that occur as the tau and the amyloid proteins migrate from one part of the brain to another, and that is how I learned about my father aiming the golf club in the wrong direction. One of my father's golf companions saw my dad do this strange thing and then told my mother, who later told me. Hearing about behavior implies, by definition, at least one degree of separation between you and the person telling you about the behavior. However, the behavior being described is often profoundly visual. I don't see very well to begin with, even when I'm looking at something directly. This statement is both literally and metaphorically true. Even with an extremely strong prescription that tries to correct for nearsightedness and astigmatism, glasses no longer make my vision 20/20. And I have already talked about not seeing my father's tears at the San Francisco Airport for what they were.

The most jaw-dropping blindness on my part was the forgetting that my father was dying. He was in a nursing home, actually a series of homes, because my mother was quite rightly and empathically never satisfied with the ones he was in. She moved him from a hellhole in Lake Worth to a fancy-pants hellhole in Jupiter, with beautiful chandeliers at the entrance and the rooms with the straitjackets in the back, to another place in Plantation (whose job is it to come up with the names of these cities?), to the last place in Delray Beach. There was always a better one over the horizon, but of course that hope was a mirage given the caregiver protocols of the '90s: patient acts up, patient gets drugged, drugs wear off, patient gets restrained. Repeat until zombified.

But back to the part where I forgot my father was dying, a cognitive maneuver that even decades later leaves me reeling in its utter strangeness. Perhaps this forgetting is the very definition of denial, self-protection, and self-immolation all rolled up into one psychic hairball. Anyway, here's what I think happened. I had become so used to visiting him in nursing homes, over the decade or so that felt like a lifetime, that at some point I think I convinced myself that this was the way things were going to be, were always going to be. This was life. Looking back, I now realize it was also death. I'm pretty sure I never thought about how my father would die (maybe some people do?), but I somehow knew how he wouldn't. The start date certainly wasn't some time during his fifties and the end date wasn't seventy. And because the way he was dying wasn't the way he was supposed to, even though exactly how he was supposed to die remained an unanswered and unposed question, I refused to acknowledge fully what was happening. I say fully because on the margins of consciousness, I knew. But I could only know for a second or two and then the knowing had to stop. Therefore (to use a word that denotes logic, even though the thought process I am describing seems crazy), as he was getting older, I managed to lose track of the passage of time. His sickness froze him in time and paralyzed me. Oddly, I could still do my academic work; in fact, I thrived. The paralysis was localized, but it went to the deepest part of me. So even as his death was happening, I didn't know it, grasp it, grieve it. Turns out, I had given myself an anesthetic that has taken about thirty years to wear off.

How I pulled off this mental magic trick—to separate my father's life in nursing homes from his impending death—still puzzles me. Let me try to explain it again. My father's battle with early-onset Alzheimer's went on for so long that I think I just thought it would keep going forever—why stop at ten years?—even though I wanted it to end so that his suffering would be over. Because his dying seemed to inhabit a continual state of deferral, I deferred acknowledging the inevitable fact of his death. I also postponed grieving the little deaths that laid the groundwork for the final one. This was a big mistake.

I remember asking myself how to grieve for an illness that could take many, many years to undo a body—and my father's was so healthy? The rational part of me (or was this the irrational part?) said I needed to pace myself. If he forgot how to load film into a camera, and I allowed myself to feel the full force of my sadness, what would I do when he couldn't talk to me or when he didn't know me? Plus, he wasn't dead. I kept waiting for my father to die so I could finally grieve, and then when he did, I couldn't. I remember that first session with a therapist in Pasadena. The air in the office was so thick with my guilt and grief that I couldn't speak. I had perpetually delayed my grief, having parceled it out like T. S. Eliot's J. Alfred Prufrock parcels out life, "I have measured out my life with coffee spoons." All I knew was postponement. When the end was near and my brother called me in California to say Dad was dying and I needed to come to Florida to say goodbye once and for all, I was shell-shocked. I had been caught between saying goodbye or not saying goodbye for so long, it was as if I were hearing the diagnosis for the first time. All those years of seeing him, and I had failed to see that he was dying.

Writing about my father's behavior and the suffering it embodied cuts to the bone because it serves as a constant reminder of my own behavior—that I was not there. And here we go again. A chapter about my father turns into a chapter about me. The mirroring that goes on when confronted with a loved one's dementia, or at least that went on in my case, is one of the weirder aspects of this weird disease. Researchers are beginning to consider this phenomenon. What happens to caregivers who spend time with a family member who has frontotemporal dementia, a disease whose hallmark is a loss of empathy? Do those caregivers lose empathy, too? Is it also the case that family members (speaking in the third person here, but *c'est moi*) of the person suffering from Alzheimer's experience a kind of contagion of forgetting? I have already talked about how I lost my memory of my healthy father as my father lost his. Surely this phenomenon also applies to depression. I sat in on a lecture Bruce gave in which he hypothesized that changes in mood are not usually responses to dementia, but rather the coming out, as it were, of the disease. He described people with Parkinson's disease as experiencing the "most ferocious" depression he had ever witnessed. Bruce is very good with words, too, and this expression has stayed with me. If your loved one is ferociously depressed, how could you not be?

I draw the line at eye trouble. That's not contagious, though certain dementias attack the occipital lobe, which is where visual circuitry lives, and my father may have had trouble seeing as the disease progressed. But if my father lost his vision toward the end of his life, I had lost mine way before. Even when I was there looking at him, I couldn't wrap my head around his illness. Learning about dementia at UCSF is my attempt to understand the illness that stole my father from me and him from himself. To look it in the eye. To think about it relentlessly. To go back thirty years and try to restore my vision (it was the not looking that actually blinded me), knowing that's a fantasy but needing to indulge it in the hopes that I can share with the world what a wonderful human being my father was, what I did and wish I had done differently when he got sick, and maybe stop punishing myself for being such a fool. But more than anything, I wish I could wrap my arms around him now and hold him as he behaved or misbehaved or whatever he was doing with his body that signified how much pain he was in. Writing this book is my attempt to do that.

•   •

Dementia is a category that encompasses a number of diseases of the brain. These include rare diseases, such as Jakob-Creutzfeldt disease (mad cow disease is a variant of this disease in animals), chronic traumatic encephalopathy (CTE), the tragic consequence of perpetually concussed football players, or amyotrophic lateral sclerosis (ALS, or Lou Gehrig's disease). Alzheimer's is the most common type of dementia, and researchers note that the risk for this illness markedly increases every decade after the age of sixty-five. By contrast, early-onset Alzheimer's is uncommon. When it strikes a person before the age of sixty-five, it can be different in presentation, course, and etiology (or original cause) of the disease. Because my father had the early-onset version of the disease, the assault on his cortex had consequences greater and faster than the typical late-onset Alzheimer's, where memory loss due to damage to the hippocampus is how the disease begins, and the illness progresses slowly. In nonscientific language, the shit hit the fan more quickly than in the typical case of Alzheimer's. His executive function capacities—writing checks, keeping track of events, knowing who he was—were taken hostage, and no amount of ransom (doctors, medicines, love, guilt) could release him from his captor because, of course, that was himself. This process differs from the memory loss that most of us associate with Alzheimer's disease. The repeated questions that were answered moments before. The not knowing at lunchtime what the person had for breakfast. Dad lost memory, too, but once the disease emerged from its prodromal phase, the obliteration of self was shockingly efficient. Picture the napalm in the opening of *Apocalypse Now* and hear the Doors' "The End" playing in the background. Something like that.

That he had early-onset Alzheimer's with the logopenic variant meant that his language problems came first, and being someone who studied language for a living, I never quite got over—as this book makes clear—that insult to my father's brain (I have learned that doctors sometimes call attacks on the brain "insults") and to my own. While focusing laser-like on that, I am now pretty sure I also missed some behaviors. Also being far away meant that the aspect of the disease to which I had the most direct access was sonic. Although short letters with typos and scratched-out words documented my father's illness, Dad's Alzheimer's was conveyed to me mostly in phone calls, short ones with short words. This is not behavior. Behavior is physical, more right side of the brain than left. More intuitive than intellectual. I am a big fan of the left hemisphere, where most of the circuitry of language lives, but the right has virtues, too. It is where creativity and feelings live. Maybe I need to go right (will that help me get right?) and remember behavior; remember being with my father and seeing his body do strange things. A particular behavior haunts me most. It is a sound—most definitely not a word—that my father made with his body. It is a sound that I not only heard, but saw. He made it with his whole body. In this chapter, I will try to connect with the right side of my brain and write that sound, which was not language but was nevertheless communicating something crucial. At the time I heard it, I didn't know what it was. But now I think I do. Looking back, hearing back, I am pretty certain it is the sound of pain. But I need to work up to writing it.

Despite not wanting to write this chapter because my gut tells me it's a hot stove that I really don't want to get close to, I understand why Bruce wants me to write it. His expertise in neurology knows no bounds as he flits, with the ease and grace of an Olympic gymnast doing backflips on the balance beam, from Broca's area to Wernicke's area, where speech and language live, from white matter to gray matter, from the left side to the right. His passion, though, is the seemingly inexplicable behavior of people with dementia, particularly frontotemporal dementia with the behavioral variant. Inabilities to empathize and to experience shame are two primary presentations of this disease. A loving husband laughs at his wife, who cries during a doctor's visit when describing how he is no longer the person she once knew. A once well-manicured woman picks through a garbage pail, eating scraps of leftover food and drinking from a found can the remnants of Mountain Dew. During a physical exam, a man is asked to hold up his arms with palms raised toward the ceiling and after a few seconds gives the doctor the finger, actually two. The middle finger on each hand.

My father didn't do these things. Or maybe he did, but I didn't see them. Here are some behaviors I didn't witness firsthand but heard about.

I was told that my mother decided that she couldn't take it anymore when my father started spreading his feces all over the bathroom walls.

I was told that he pulled the sink out of the wall at the nursing home. I remember being proud of his rage. If he could be angry and he was still that strong, he was still there, and it confirmed my own need to be enraged. I remember hearing about this incident and immediately thinking of Dylan Thomas's poem "Do Not Go Gentle into That Good Night," as I pictured my father battling it out with the sink, with the disease. But having learned at UCSF about the right ways and the wrong ways of caregiving, I know now that he was probably battling on many fronts, not just the disease. He was angry at the noises in the nursing home, the drugs, the showers from strangers, the external prison he was in, as well as the internal one. Part of me wishes he had gone gently, but that's not who he was—even in death.

I was told that he had sundowners. I remember the moment vividly. It was over lunch at a restaurant in Bethesda, Maryland with my mother and sister. The word "sundowners" was woven into the conversation in such a way that there was an assumption that I knew what it was, even though no one had told me. Which is why I erupted, ever the potty-mouthed woman once I embraced the power that comes with the effective use of a well-placed curse word, and asked, "What the fuck is sundowners?" I thought my father had another disease about which I had not been told. As if Alzheimer's weren't enough. After being told to quiet down and calm down and not say "fuck" so loud and in public, I was informed that sundowners is a not uncommon condition that people with Alzheimer's sometimes have, and that it happens when day turns into night. As if the days and nights weren't hard enough for my dad, the transition from one to the other was especially tough. I have since learned that the setting of the sun can lead to agitation, anxiety, and aggressive behaviors. I wonder if my dad pulled out the sink at around 5 p.m. I wonder what else he was doing when the sun went down.

I was told my father flipped out because my sister was driving. She had had her license for decades, but my father thought she was a child.

I was told he was straitjacketed. This makes me crazy.

Bruce has explained to me that despite the fact that Alzheimer's disease begins in a specific region of the brain, probably even within a single cell, at a certain point the whole brain surrenders. Thus, the neat categories into which one might put symptoms in the earlier stages of a person's illness eventually make no sense. People with Alzheimer's disease can look like people with Parkinson's, later in the illness. And so my father shuffled and shook and did not have the muscle strength to hold me tight like he used to when I was little. They can look like people with frontotemporal dementia and unashamedly wipe their excrement all over the bathroom. People with Alzheimer's may end up hallucinating, a typical and horrific indicator of Lewy body disease. Not the Lucy-in-the-sky kind of hallucination, but the sort that scares the hell out of you. The kind that ends up putting you in a straitjacket.

I have to wonder, though, if some of my father's behaviors—especially those that manifested themselves in the nursing homes—were the result of the disease or the medicines he was given to relieve its symptoms. This is the generous reading; that pulling out the sink signified the disease gone wild and not my father's reaction to an antipsychotic drug used to treat schizophrenia that was making him go crazy. Also generous is the notion that the medicines were intended as relief; that the sleeping pills were actually meant to help him sleep as opposed to knocking him out and turning him into a zombie. The more cynical version, and the one I subscribe to, is that the doctors at the time didn't fully understand the implications of what they were doing, and the nursing homes wanted its inmates to be quiet. To behave. Whatever it took. Antipsychotics. Antianxiety medications. Sleeping pills. Straitjackets. In this reading, the medicines weren't about relieving my father but instead relieving the nursing home.

My father's agitation agitated the nursing home. Agitation seems to be the code word that gets the pharmacological ball rolling. Agitation equals misbehavior. If you get called agitated, you're in trouble. The dilemma of being labeled "agitated" resonates with me. As a child, my mother sometimes called me *"broygus"* (pronounced phonetically, emphasis on the "broy"). According to the *Jewish English Lexicon*, it means angry or annoyed. Cranky, if you will. Like broygus, cranky is one of those heads-

I-win-tails-you-lose words. My own experience taught me that to be broygus was to disagree and therefore to be disagreeable. At the time, I didn't question how the verb immediately became an adjective. Anyway, this onomatopoeic Yiddish word, and there are so many that I love (think *bubelah*, *kvelling*, *verklempt*), could be weaponized in any number of contexts. My mother and I might be clothes shopping and I didn't want to try on the outfit she liked. Maybe I didn't want to have dinner with my aunt and uncle. Maybe I didn't want to make my bed. Often, I would cry in response to being called broygus, which of course only confirmed the perspective of the person hurling that epithet at me. The point is that once called broygus, you were doomed. If you conceded that you were, you were. If you objected that you weren't, that was just more evidence that you were.

Agitation works similarly, but the structural analogy ends there. In the nursing home setting, the stakes couldn't be higher. You get medicine for being agitated, and if you put up a fuss and don't want to take the medicine, you just get more because the refusal to take medicine is a sign that you're agitated. Before you know it, the tranquilizer prescription that is listed as a PRN, the abbreviation for the Latin *pre re nata*, which loosely means "as needed," becomes needed, and you're zonked out on Klonopin. To which I ask, "Cui bono?," which loosely translates to, "Who is benefiting from this?" Other examples of agitation include a refusal to shower or an unwillingness to leave one's room or a desire to leave the nursing home and go home. One can, however, put these alleged misbehaviors more positively, and redefine agitation as a normative aspect of the human condition. Think about how you feel at the DMV or when a person gets in the fifteen-items-or-less line at the grocery store when their cart is overflowing. The experience of agitation transgresses the dividing line between illness and health. No longer medicalized, agitation means a desire to hasten one's death by refusing more pills. It signals a desire to have control over one's body as opposed to having a stranger touch you in the shower. Maybe it means a desire to be left alone in order to tune out what is often the din of a nursing home environment. Putting it this way, wanting to leave that environment seems like the definition of rationality.

The approach now recommended by experts at UCSF is the opposite of what my father endured. Pharmaceutical interventions are a last resort. Try music if the person is upset. I think listening to Frank Sinatra might well have calmed down my father when he was frightened. Try specially trained dogs. I am certain that my father would have relaxed if emotional support animals had been a resource. Not only would he have been comforted in the moment, but he also may have remembered being comforted in the past by Tocca. Intergenerational approaches to caregiving are gaining traction, with benefits seeming to accrue to the young as well as the old. Studies have shown that elders experience increased cognitive well-being, and younger people feel more valued, more connected. My brother is working on how Maria Montessori's approaches can be implemented in order to ease the everyday challenges faced by people with dementia and their caregivers. And when it comes to the use of drugs, rather than knocking people out with sedatives, the most up-to-date science of caregiving suggests that the best course of action involves keeping people awake during the day so that the chances of sleeping during the night improve. Seems like a no-brainer. Haldol, the antipsychotic used to treat schizophrenia, and which my father took, should rarely be given to people with Alzheimer's. Rather than helping, it often makes the situation worse. And straitjackets should only be used in rare cases where the person might harm herself or others.

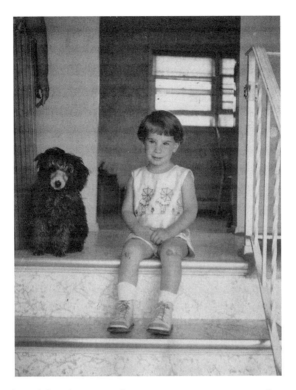

Cindy with her dog, Tocca, in Verona, New Jersey (year unknown)

But before my father ended up in his first nursing home and before he became big pharma's dream come true, he was metamorphosing into someone else. I remember a couple of behaviors that felt more like surprise attacks from an invisible enemy during one fall visit in the 1980s to Bethesda, where my sister and her family lived, and my parents spent a lot of time. This may or may not have been the same trip when I learned my father had sundowners. It may or may not have been the same trip where I showed him how to cut a cantaloupe.

My sister had moved heaven and earth to get my father into an Alzheimer's clinical trial at the National Institutes of Health, which was located a few miles from her home. Although Dad was too far into the illness—he had moved out of what I now know is called the mild cognitive impairment phase, where everyday tasks are harder to complete, but not impossible as they eventually will be—she somehow managed to persuade the researchers to let my father in. My parents left their place in Florida and rented a two-bedroom apartment close to NIH. I flew in from Berkeley.

I can remember three things about that time in Maryland in the fall of 1986. The first and best, as in happiest, memory is my father's laughter. He and I took a walk around the lush grounds of the apartment complex. It was the afternoon and it had rained the day before and the sky was clear and the air was crisp, not unlike one of the fall days in New Jersey when we would go to Verona High School on a Saturday afternoon and watch the Verona Hillbillies play and usually lose a football game. Something in one of the ponds that dotted the grounds where we were walking—I can't remember what it was—captured my attention. While Dad stayed several feet away from the water, I approached the edge of the pond only to lose my balance and slip in the mud and into the water. Dad smiled and laughed. Me too. I had always been a klutz, and my falling confirmed the fact that some things hadn't changed. The depression, my father's and my own, lifted for an instant. Such a small moment to remember, but it was the highlight of the visit.

The second thing I remember—and this is a behavior—is waking up in the middle of the night, having set up quarters in the second bedroom of the Bethesda apartment, and seeing my father standing over the bed and looking at me. No, staring at me with a concentration that I recall taking note of and being surprised by. Before I go any further with this memory, I should say that my father never slept very well. Where he slept best was downstairs in our split-level house while watching television in his favorite burnt-red leather chair that had an ottoman to match. On the weekends, when he would happily descend the stairs into the loving arms of the chair, with our dog Tocca on his lap and me squished next to him in the chair, I would make fun of his journey from eyes wide open watching Jack Nicklaus, the Tiger Woods of the 1960s and '70s, make a birdie, to eyes at half-mast taking in the dulcet sounds of NBC announcer Jim McKay's commentary, to eyes fully closed as Jack received one of his six Master's tournament trophies.

As a little kid, I always found it intriguing that Jim, or Pat Summerall, spoke in hushed tones. It wasn't like they were on the golf course and their voices would have distracted the players. I guess they were modeling the quiet that was expected of the viewers who were actually there. I can recall the announcers for the bowling competitions similarly using what we would now call their inside voices. Maybe it was a media strategy to amp up, or more precisely, create some anticipatory drama around bowling. The clash of the pins contrasted nicely with the hush of the viewers. In any case, the announcers' whispers, whether on the putting green or in the alley, acted as lullabies for my father, and I would try hard to refrain from giggling when Dad would start snoring.

Maybe his insomnia was an early warning sign of things to come? Or maybe it laid the groundwork for that first cell to go rogue, making the brain vulnerable to attack? Sleep, it turns out, is crucial for the well-being of the brain, as well as for physical health. We all know that we feel better after a good night's rest, and one of the most effective torture techniques involves disrupting a person's sleep. But it may be that brains require sleep to remain healthy. Scientists think that we sleep in order to rid our brains of the amyloid proteins that we all have. Without good sleep, the toxins can't be evacuated, and they build up. Conversely, scientists also think that insomnia may be a sign, an effect rather than a cause, that all is not well in the brain. Bad sleep might mean that toxins have accumulated (see Bruce's description in our next chapter). With these hypotheses, I think back to my parent's bedroom in Lake Worth. It looked like a theater of war. My father did not need someone to torture him. His brain took care of it. I see the bed in the morning. Sheets are draped over the headboard. Blankets crumpled up and strewn all over the place. Some pillows lie where they belong, others askew at the foot of the bed with pillowcases half-on half-off. The mattress is partly on the box spring, the rest of it on a diagonal touching the carpeting. Lord knows how and where my mother slept. Maybe this was another reason she decided she couldn't take it anymore and put my father in a nursing home.

When I was sleeping in Bethesda near NIH, the room was dark, and I felt a presence that woke me up. Unlike my usual fraidy-cat reaction to unexpected things that happen in the dark, I acted as if the whole situation were normal and remember saying hello to my dad and taking his hand and walking him back into his bedroom. On the one hand, I am now pretty convinced that my father was staring at me because he didn't know who I was. On the other hand, maybe he knew who I was and wanted to take me in as much as possible. Kind of like building credit or memory so that it would take longer for him to forget who I was. And on the one hand, I wish I had asked him why he was staring at me. Maybe he would have told me how much he loved me and missed me. Maybe he would have told me that he didn't know me, and we could have cried about that together. I don't think there is an on the other hand. I never cried with my father about his disease. My heart is broken by this non-memory.

The other memory of this visit leads me to think that my father had bigger fish to fry than perhaps not knowing me or indulging me in just one good cry that I could hold onto so that he would know, even though he would forget it, how utterly devastated I was that he was sick. I'm pretty sure he didn't know himself. I say this based on a behavior I saw. It was in that apartment in Bethesda that I started noticing how often Dad took out his wallet and put it back again. In between the taking out and the putting back was another step. He would pull out his driver's license, which he retained despite not being able to drive anymore, his Medicare card, and his credit card. His hand shook a little bit putting the plastic cards back in place—maybe the beginnings of Parkinson's?—but I focused less on that and more on the possibility that he was looking for his name, his identity, for who he was. The first time he did this, I thought he was checking to see if he had misplaced one of the cards and wanted to make sure it was there. We all do that. The second time, I knew it was more than that, because he had checked his wallet only minutes before. The third and fourth and fifth times, I realized I was looking at something I didn't want to see. And here I am faced with another one of my behaviors in the face of my father's behavior that brings me to my knees. Instead of gently asking him if I could help him find something or instead of simply hugging him because he was feeling so unanchored in the universe, I did a really stupid thing. I retreated to my intellect.

What did this mental double Axel, triple Lutz look like? I need to back up for a moment and provide some academic context in order to make clear how my mind translated the incomprehensibility of my father's illness into a framework that I understood, could control, and wasn't afraid of; in other words, a framework that was the opposite of a disease that defied explanation, wouldn't be controlled, and frightened me to death. I write this, and it is clear that I was out of my mind. Here it goes.

If you were lucky enough to be studying to get a PhD in literature in the 1980s, you would have taken at least one class in literary theory where course syllabi included titles such as "Is there a text in this class?" or "What is an author?" or "The death of the author." The idea is that what a reader had always thought of as stable or real—whether that be the book she was holding or the person who wrote it—is not. The text we read is a function of the interpretations made by readers. The author is not the creator of a text, but rather a function of it. Notice the presence of an absence. The word "identity" was written as *"identity,"* and the very idea of a self was understood to be performed and under constant construction. I enjoyed questioning these aspects of literature—the text I was reading or the author of it—that had previously been taken for granted. Edgar Allan Poe, for example, had a fondness for plagiarism. Were his texts really *his* if complete paragraphs had been poached from others' writings? In the only novel Poe wrote, *The Narrative of Arthur Gordon Pym*, the narrator and fictional Pym refers to Poe, the real author, as the fictional character! My mind luxuriated in the breakdown of fiction and nonfiction; in the reversibility of Pym and Poe; in the release from the ball and chain of self. Theory was heady and fun.

In Bethesda, I witnessed my father being released from himself, and it wasn't fun. It made me nauseous, watching his identity become an *identity.* And as I watched my father look for himself in his wallet, my mind broke down and broke apart. Emily Dickinson beautifully describes this mental state in her poem "I felt a Funeral, in my Brain." Dickinson's poetic funeral is noisy, with its "treading – treading" and its "beating – beating." I too heard a clanging in my head as I tried to drown out the deafening reality of what I was seeing and feeling as my dad struggled to remind himself of who he was. Fiction and poetry poured into my mind, roared into it because I couldn't bear to see or hear or accept what was happening. My father's sickness was so loud and awful and threatening to everything that I knew and loved that my response was to drown it out in order to cancel it out with competing sounds that I loved. Dickinson, Eliot, Poe.

Except there is one sound I can't obliterate, and now I am no longer going to try. We are in the nursing home in Delray Beach, and my father is unkempt. The man who was a neatnik, whose side of the bedroom was always much tidier than my mother's, whose slippers were always placed carefully beneath the night table, is disheveled. His caregiver had given him a shave days before, but I suspect he would only put up with so much grooming and so the stubble has grown back. The man who smelled of Old Spice, my father who let me put his shaving cream on my face and pretend-shave with him. His hair is oily. He is only in his sixties, but he looks about ninety, closer to his mother's age than to my mother, who was two years younger than her Jerry. His eyes are vacant at first, but when I look at him, we connect. I go in to give him a hug. He is trembling and doesn't quite know that his arms should surround me. I hold his hand and talk about nonsense that I am pretty sure he doesn't understand and then he makes that sound.

The medical word for this sound is bruxism. It's a weird word and apparently comes from the Greek, *brychein*, which means "to gnash the teeth." Turns out, I had a case of bruxism when I was little. When I was at summer camp, I apparently had such a bad habit of grinding my teeth my fellow bunkmates sometimes thought an animal had entered the cabin. I don't know or care why I had it. I want to talk about my father's case. Bruxism can signal tension, stress, anxiety, frustration, pain. People with dementia sometimes have bruxism, and certain psychiatric medicines, like the kind given to my father in the nursing homes, can worsen the condition.

Bruxism, schmuxism. Here's what my dad's looked and sounded like in those years when I went to see him in the nursing home with my mother, and then we would leave after the too-short visit and want to die but would go shopping or out to eat instead. His eyes look frightened, and he starts breathing hard. His lips are open, and his front teeth touch the bottom teeth, and then a whooshing sound comes out that goes "shhhh," "shhhh." I am not satisfied with that description because "shhhh" sounds too much like shush, and that's not what I hear. It is loud, and Emily Dickinson is quiet now, and I can hear it and do it with my own lips and mouth and try to translate the sound I am remembering and making. Dad is scared. His body doesn't know what to do with itself. His chest heaves up and down. His mouth is slightly open, his tongue trapped in place, and he makes a "sh" sound that contains remnants of saliva and he keeps repeating it. The sound is all breath, with no voice behind it or within it. And there is a sort of elongated vowel sound at the end of the "sh." It's an "eeee." His face is pained. His body is taut and at its wit's end. The sound is pain. It is the sound of my father's dementia.

The Neglected and Poorly Understood

Progressive cognitive and functional decline leading to dementia is a definitional feature of Alzheimer's disease. In fact, nearly all of the neurodegenerative conditions, including Alzheimer's disease, are associated with changes in cognition, movement, and behavior. Cognition and movement have been systematically analyzed in the setting of dementia, facilitating our understanding of how we speak, comprehend, name, remember, plan, multitask, generate ideas, navigate space, and carry out complex movements. By contrast, until recently, the clinical patterns and anatomic substrates of behavior in dementia were neglected and poorly understood.

The reason for this neglect is complex and multifactorial, but it says a lot about how science and society have dichotomized cognition and movement as localized to the brain, while mood and behavior have been considered through social and psychological paradigms. When someone has trouble with speaking, remembering, or moving, it does not take long before they are referred to a physician with the expectation that they suffer from a disorder of the brain. By contrast, if the same person had exhibited a mood disorder, psychosis, disinhibition, or profound apathy as the first manifestation of a neurodegenerative condition, a neurological evaluation would rarely be considered. In fact, more than one-half of the people (70 percent of the women) in my UCSF patient population with frontotemporal dementia are first diagnosed as suffering from a psychiatric condition. Often, they bounce from one system to another before the true cause for their behavioral changes is determined.

There are historical reasons for this gap. In the beginnings of psychiatry and neurology in the late 1800s, the two fields were fused into a single entity. When many of the important discoveries from Pick, Fischer, Alzheimer, Lewy, and Jakob were made, there were neuropsychiatrists who studied the brain and behavior. Yet, by the turn of the twentieth century, the fields began to split, leaving neurology to the study of conditions for which there was a known brain abnormality, like epilepsy, stroke, or brain tumor, and psychiatry was left to the description of behaviors/disorders where brain localization was not considered possible, like schizophrenia, bipolar disorder, and depression. Of note, neurodegenerative disorders such as Alzheimer's disease, frontotemporal dementia, Parkinson's disease, Lou Gehrig's disease—fell in between the two fields and still do.

The consequence for this split was profound. Psychiatry moved to the study of the unconscious and to the description of what people did and felt, while neurology eliminated the study of feelings (depression, anxiety, guilt) or behavior as a domain of the specialty. Ultimately, this proved problematic for both fields, as psychiatry systematically abandoned brain anatomy and physiology as a way to understand the cause and potential treatment for their conditions, and neurology eliminated evaluation of the phenomenology of behavior, ignoring the 30 percent of the brain that makes up the cerebral cortex.

This split was especially problematic for the neurodegenerative conditions in which microscopic anatomic lesions were the basis for symptoms. Until recently, these subtle lesions could not be measured during life, and many symptoms were neglected. This is changing, and researchers are demonstrating that parkinsonian conditions and Alzheimer's disease often begin as a mood, anxiety, or sleep disorder due to degeneration in the brainstem and other deep brain structures where mood, anxiety, and sleep are generated and controlled. Similarly, the socially inappropriate behaviors (disinhibition), apathy, compulsions, and overeating seen in frontotemporal dementia are due to degeneration in the frontal and anterior temporal lobes and the basal ganglia regions critical for the social modulation of behavior. Hence, in a disease with well-established anatomy, previously healthy people eat food off of others' plates, make inappropriate comments at meetings, touch or even caress strangers, or collect and drink soda from garbage cans. Further, through the work of Jessica Jimenez and Mazen Kheirbek at UCSF, we have learned that in mice there are cells in the hippocampus that connect with deep structures in the hypothalamus that are responsible for the control of anxiety. This finding puts the presence of anxiety, irritability, and agitation in Alzheimer's disease in a new light. Maybe anxiety is more than just a reaction to memory loss. Maybe it is actually a manifestation of hippocampal dysfunction. Measuring mood and behavior is critical for early diagnosis and eventually early treatment. Also, these changes have their own specific therapies. Further, accepting that abnormal behaviors are driven by changes in the brain takes pressure off of families, who blame themselves or the person who is sick for what has happened.

Jerry's illness began with language and other cognitive symptoms, but he also developed sadness, irritability, agitation, and bruxism at various stages of his illness. Understanding how much of Jerry's grief, irritability, and agitation was a reaction to the circumstances of his predicament and how much was due to brain changes related to Alzheimer's disease is hard to know. We tend to interpret behavior through our own unique lenses and biases. For a psychologist, Jerry's depression might be interpreted as the release of long-suppressed resentment toward his parents for lack of nurturance. For an empathic daughter or son, the sadness could be explained as due to Jerry's awareness of his cognitive losses, while for a child or relative who was less sympathetic to Jerry during life, the irritability might be described as longstanding and just an exaggeration of his underlying baseline negative traits. For someone who mistrusts medications, the behaviors could be explained by the medications that were prescribed to manage Jerry's behavior. Finally, for a fanatically religious person, the psychiatric symptoms might be due to Jerry's imperfect relationship with God. Even within a single family, the behaviors of Alzheimer's disease can be seen through a multitude of different perspectives.

Indeed, these ways of seeing and explaining behavior in the setting of dementia can be like the movie *Rashomon* from Japanese filmmaker Akira Kurosawa, where witnesses to, participants in, and victims of a crime all describe a different version of what happened. Alzheimer's disease is a crime against the brain, but which of these multitudes of interpretations is most accurate? Yes, we all have unconscious conflicts, carry an unpleasant trait or two, respond badly to psychoactive medications, have imperfect relations with our maker, and, even in the setting of dementia, can generate self-reflection about the impact of our condition upon a sense of well-being. Yet, as a behavioral neurologist, I question whether any of the explanations truly capture the whys and whats of behavior in dementia. It is telling that we never evoke psychological hypotheses when someone develops a problem with memory or language. Usually we accept—it's the brain.

My teacher Frank Benson had a simple dictum, "A change in personality or a well-established pattern of behavior represents a change in the brain." Early in his illness, Jerry developed a somber sadness, although we never hear about serious discussion with Cindy regarding his worries or hopes for his or her future like we might have if he had suffered from a terminal cancer that did not affect his brain. Rather, all the reflection is Cindy. There are probably many reasons that this discussion didn't take place, including a tendency in the 1980s and '90s for families to make the discussion of dementia a taboo. I also wonder whether there was some—what we neurologists call anosognosia—lack of awareness or denial of illness. Anosognosia often accompanies neurodegenerative conditions. This is particularly true of the behavioral variant of frontotemporal dementia, but it also happens with Alzheimer's disease. We know from the literature on stroke that anosognosia is common with disease on the right side of the brain whether frontal, temporal, or parietal. From Cindy's eloquent story, we know that Jerry had both left and right parietal lobe dysfunction.

Denial is extremely frustrating for families and loved ones. It prevents honest dialogue and can lead patients to refuse to take medications, to insist that they can drive well and can manage with bills and legal documents when they can't. I would expect that some element of anosognosia followed Jerry throughout the course of his Alzheimer's disease. While this denial is part of the burden of the disease, it may be that it blunts the tragedy of the illness for the patient, who continues to believe that their life is normal, or at least not that disabled.

Later we hear that there were episodes of agitation, evidenced by a sink torn out of the wall. There is a tendency to smile in admiration, as we think of Jerry protesting his state with this deed of defiance. Yet, this story is a marker of how difficult, possibly even threatening, Jerry might have been for staff once his illness had progressed. Delusions, hallucinations, irritability, and agitation often take over in the mid-to-later stages of Alzheimer's disease, as higher cognitive functions are erased and more basic behaviors, programmed in the brain for attack and defense, take over.

Hence, the onslaught of medications that Jerry received. Cindy is right; often the medications are prescribed to keep the patient manageable without concern for their negative impact upon awareness, drive, cognition, and movement. These medications can be lethal. Almost certainly, Jerry was overmedicated, and in the 1980s and '90s, antipsychotics were grossly overprescribed. Even today they are overprescribed. Unfortunately, the science for the treatment of behavior in dementia is in its infancy, and we have learned that most of the time the medications that we use are ineffective or worse. It's all trial and error, and the trial often fails. Too often we accept blunting of cognition, movement, and behavior as an alternative to more subtle medication regimens. Sometimes there is no choice.

We tend to forget that a remarkable patriarch like Jerry Weinstein brings huge pride to a family, and so much of their identity comes from his intelligence, nurturance, and overall status within society. The whooshing sound that Jerry begins to make in the later stages of his illness is sadly real, unbearably real. We all understand how hard it is and must have been for Cindy to see and experience a grand man brought to this level. The sound is a symbol of Jerry's suffering, and it also represents a degradation of his social presence in the world. When someone like Cindy, with deep empathy and admiration for her father, watches such a devastating decline in a parent, it shakes their world, and shakes it forever. The tragedy makes even the most brilliantly written play or novel pale in comparison.

In 2004, my father, uniquely generous, original, and humanistic, an academic psychiatrist devoted to the underserved, developed a malignant right parietal brain tumor. He was in his late seventies, and at the time of the diagnosis, his creativity and vitality were still extraordinary, almost superhuman. He was the head of Psychiatry at Harbor-UCLA Medical Center and oversaw mental health for the county of Los Angeles. Dad had a multitude of friends who adored him, people he had helped and mentored. Many were crushed by this diagnosis, and some were eager to help. Slightly dispiriting and surprising to Dad, other "friends" quickly evaporated when it became clear that he was going to lose power. Me, Mom, my brother and sister, our large extended family, and a few friends became his support team. After Dad got very sick, we hired Larry, a caregiver from the Philippines to help. For Dad's physicians, the hospice team, etc., well, it still brings a bitter taste to my mouth. I don't think that I have ever forgiven them.

After the diagnosis, for a few months, my father continued with his characteristic buoyant optimism and positivity. He frantically set his affairs in order while continuing to work. Then, he started to decline, physically, and there were subtle mental changes as well. I realized that Dad was no longer going to be my major source of advice, optimism, and good spirit. Dad became quiet, even somber. I think that there was some depression, although I don't really know. He never, ever complained of his mood or his situation. Meals, typically a cause for celebration and vibrant discussion, were quiet except for pleasantries exchanged about the food. A dark cloud hovered over Mom and Dad's beautiful little cottage that sat on a cliff overlooking the ocean in San Pedro, California. Soon Dad was unable to use the left side of his body and required a wheelchair.

I remember a sunny Saturday morning when Mom, Dad, and I went to Mom's hair stylist in Redondo Beach. It felt unnatural wheeling Father into a beauty shop. We nodded and offered greetings. After quick glances at Dad, all of the attention was directed toward me. From the largest presence in any room, Dad was now invisible.

I rolled Dad out from the beauty shop down toward the ocean, a place where he and Mom had lived and a place that they loved. The trip was silent. I was deep in thought, and Dad just looked straight ahead. As we approached the ocean I began to cry, bawl. It went on for several minutes. I touched Dad. It was unusual for me to touch Dad, and we never hugged. He looked back but remained silent. We rolled back to the beauty shop to pick up Mom. My tears represented an awareness that a world that I loved was changing forever. It did.

I never saw Dad cry, and I don't cry often either. In fact, it has happened only a few times in my adult life. At the age of eighteen in 1967, my mother's father, Herman, was dying, and my girlfriend came to visit me at college. We had been together from my sophomore year in high school, but we were beginning to drift apart. During our discussion about my grandfather, I started to cry. I cried so hard that my nose bled all over the green-gray dormitory carpet. We tried to rub out the blood with paper towels from the bathroom, but I am sure that the stains were there for the life of the carpet. In 1985, my brother and I flew back to Indiana from Los Angeles to visit my father's dad, William Miller, who was dying with a variety of conditions. Grandpa Bill had paid for my college science training before I pursued medical school. We were close. At the time, I was finishing a fellowship and faced huge uncertainty in my life. We were sitting backward in the front row of a flight and I was listening to Dionne Warwick sing "That's What Friends Are For," and the tears burst forth. The whole front of the plane seemed fixed upon me. My brother looked at me aghast.

Crying is a brainstem reflex orchestrated by the autonomic nervous system. The muscles of the face contract in a specific pattern, tears are released from the lacrimal gland, heart rate and sweating increase, and breathing decreases. Often, after crying, there is a resolution of grief. While crying is a basic reflex, the triggers are complex and reflect the vast expanse of our cortex. My tears are triggered by long periods of stress thinking about the loss of a loved one who has been a central part of my life. I cry about lost love, lost loved ones, and death. In "Crying," Roy Orbison sings about a lost love, "Then you said so long / Left me standing all alone / Alone and crying."

With age come slowly progressive diseases of the brain. We lose our protectors, people who have shaped us the most, like spouses, parents, grandparents, friends, sometimes even children. These are important people in our universe, a universe that lies in our brain. We know that this same process of deterioration and loss can happen to us. I understand how the sound that Jerry made became the trigger and catalyst for Cindy to forget. Perhaps if she had cried, it would have softened the blow, and she would have been able to remember earlier. It was the end of a chapter in her universe. I am lucky, we are all lucky, that she dared to remember. We all have to remember.

· 5 ·

Memory

In Memoriam: Jerry Weinstein

Most novels are told retrospectively; that is, they are narrated in the past tense. For example, various experiences happen to Charles Dickens's David Copperfield or Oliver Twist, and the narrator looks back (sometimes the narrator is the protagonist, or main character) and tells us what they were. The plot is then made up of key events that take place in the protagonist's youth that lead to choices made or not made that create the person about whom we are reading. These events can and usually do include losing one or both parents (or losing and then finding one, as is the case in *Oliver Twist*); getting adopted; getting educated; falling in and out of love. You know, having a life. These stories about a protagonist growing up and wending her way in the world make up a literary genre called the bildungsroman. For this genre to work, it is essential that someone—the protagonist, the narrator—remember the past. My father lost his ability to narrate his past when he lost his ability to remember and to speak. Alzheimer's was a kind of un-building. There must be many stories about his past and our shared past that he would have told me if he hadn't gotten sick, and those events died when my father died. I lost the past, too. The past we shared before he lost those things. I'm going to see if I can find it.

Before my father became ill, the highlights of my own bildungsroman, or journey from childhood to adulthood, would have included the following: years in summer camp, years taking piano lessons, trips to Florida to visit my Grandma Sarah, a couple of solo adventures as a young teenager to Los Angeles to visit cousins, and a bout with anorexia. Alongside these events would be the threads that led me to loving letters and words and, by extension, literature. The days playing Scrabble after school with my mother. The hours working on the *New York Times* crossword puzzle, especially on Sundays, well before the advent of Google, which meant a whole day of the weekend spent with a dictionary, as well as a host of encyclopedias and atlases which surely have little relation to our present-day world. My mother's insistence that I read Dickens before Erich Segal's *Love Story*. The two books on the shelf behind the toilet in my brother's bathroom—*The Hobbit*, which I could never get through, and *The Catcher in the Rye*, which I could. Going to the Princeton University library, where my sister went to college, and doing junior high school homework (she is almost nine years older than I) surrounded by books and the hush of people reading them and loving that. Spending six weeks at the Phillips Academy Andover summer session, during which time I took two literature classes and read twelve books and knowing this is what I want to do with my life. I was sixteen that summer, and that fall I read *Moby-Dick* for the first time (who writes a book about a one-legged captain chasing a white whale?), and my brother introduced me to Bob Dylan (who writes a rock-and-roll song about a leopard-skin pillbox hat?), and things were never the same.

Literature was a vehicle for trying on identities, for positioning myself in relation to others, for figuring out what world I wanted to occupy while reading about what alternative worlds were out there. In advanced placement English, Sinclair Lewis's *Main Street*—a story about the trappings of suburbia—gave me the language to understand how boring my hometown of Verona, New Jersey, was. I read Albert Camus's *The Stranger*, about the (seemingly) senseless murder of an Arab by a French Algerian, and became an existentialist. I read Kate Chopin's *The Awakening*, the story of a wealthy but deeply dissatisfied married woman who ends up walking into the ocean and never coming back, and discovered feminism, nineteenth-century style. Eugène Ionesco's play *Rhinoceros*, where rhinoceri run around a small town, turned me into an absurdist. By the time college started, I was deeply and forever in love with literature. Thus, when one of my professors thundered the Greek word *"anagnorosis,"* which means realization or epiphany, in his lecture on Homer's *Iliad*, I was like one of those swooning, ecstatic girls in the video montages of the Beatles when they're singing "I Want to Hold Your Hand."

This was before my father was diagnosed with Alzheimer's disease. I loved literature before that. I say this because it is hard to remember what came before. The fact is that when my father got sick and couldn't have a conversation with me anymore, on the phone or in person, I felt like everything that came before got wiped out and anything that came after would disappear, and the only question was how long it would take to not remember. It was some deranged race against time. How does one race to remember? What does that even mean? Racing is going forward; remembering is going backward. In practical terms, it meant that there could be nothing new—no new memories to create—because he couldn't hold onto what was happening in the present, let alone the future, and so there was only the past. And Alzheimer's was making a hash of that.

My analogy for a brain being attacked by Alzheimer's is nothing original and probably medically wrong. I know scientists see plaques and tangles. I imagine an encroaching darkness that culminates in blankness, something more like the macular degeneration that my nana had. That condition of diminishing eyesight begins by attacking the center of one's vision and then radiates outward until the peripheral damage is complete. As this happens, things just get blurrier and blurrier, until you can't see. The transcendental philosopher Ralph Waldo Emerson writes in his 1836 essay "Nature" about how being "in the woods, we return to reason and faith." He continues, "There I feel that nothing can befall me in life,–no disgrace, no calamity, (leaving me my eyes,) which nature cannot repair." My theory, based on a penchant for finding structural similarities whether they exist or not, is that what macular degeneration does to the eyes, Alzheimer's does to the mind. If this is true and if given a choice between losing sight or cognition (are you there God, it's me Cindy?), I'll take the former.

But back to that analogy. In the early eighteenth century, the philosopher John Locke came up with the image of the mind as a tabula rasa, or a blank slate, waiting to be filled in by experience and knowledge that would become the life of the person, their memory. Because I am a teacher (and was born in 1960), I imagine a chalkboard. Think about being in school and walking into the classroom where a math or an English class has just been taught. The board hasn't been erased yet. There are signs and words all over. My dad's mind was like a chalkboard (or whiteboard) filled with equations and words— memories—and Alzheimer's came along and took an eraser to each number, each word, each memory. It would take many years to get rid of the writing (the memories, the mental and physical life). And as if that weren't grotesque enough, the disease had a nasty habit of screwing with the numbers and the words before sending them into oblivion. Prior to complete erasure, letters would be moved around, and words would be misspelled. Or the math would be wrong. In the early days / early years of the disease, my father knew things were wrong and therefore was daily, by the minute, confronted with the fact of his diminishing capacities. He would pleadingly ask, "What is wrong with me?" or declare, "Something is wrong with me." But we couldn't tell him what it was, and even if we had, he probably wouldn't have been able to hang onto that fact long enough to kill himself.

Enough agony for everyone. Sometimes the words or the numbers would look right, add up for a moment (has the disease taken some time off?), but no. Just a temporary break in the assault to delete all things. Fifty-plus years to write on the board. Fifteen, give or take, to erase everything on it. The emptiness that is left is no tabula rasa, though, waiting for another round of memories to be created. No, this tabula has had its legs yanked out, its top smashed to bits, and has been rendered incapable of being written on. As with deforestation, no trees can grow again. Like a garden hose with a hole in it, the water can't get to its destination, leaving what was once alive starving and desiccated. What begins as an interesting philosophical notion of the mind as a tabula rasa, a blank mind that will become that person's life, their memory, has the tables turned on itself. This is a mind made blank over time. How much time is anyone's guess.

At the same time as my father was losing his memory, I kind of lost mine, too. Not everything of course. I could recall the time when, in my sister's house, I showed my father how to cut a cantaloupe. He was standing around in the kitchen, wanting to help with preparing the food, but he had forgotten how to use a knife. My mother commended me on my patience and ingenuity because I had found something that Dad could do.

I remember one day sitting on the counter stools in Dunkin Donuts, the one in Lake Worth, when he couldn't remember what he had done the day before so we talked about what he had done decades before, and I told him what a wonderful dad he was and that would never change just because he couldn't remember things. I could access the memory of getting off the plane in the West Palm Beach airport, feeling like an elephant was sitting on my chest, girding myself for the lack of recognition that was coming any day now. It didn't come that day. And of course, I remembered the things that were my lifeline or seemed that way at the time: authors, dates, characters, the argument of my dissertation, blah, blah, blah. The more I threw myself into the lives and plots of dead authors and their make-believe characters, the further my grief about my father receded. I thought that was good because the pain didn't feel quite so bad.

But actually, what got erased was my memory of my father pre-Alzheimer's. Let's call it, for irony or perversity's sake, B.A.D.—Before Alzheimer's Disease. This is perverse because I remember many of the bad things extraordinarily well. It's the good things, the things Before Alzheimer's Disease, that have been difficult to access. And with good reason. I put them away so I couldn't find them and remember how much they meant to me. I buried these treasures because they were both precious and gone. The trauma of losing my father in this way first made me unable and then made me unwilling to remember what I had lost. I ran for cover in literature. Over the years, literature (and words) gave me (and continues to give me) both an escape hatch and a vocabulary to take on the trauma of losing my father and not go completely crazy. With novels, I could immerse myself in the pleasures and the pains of other lives so I could take a break from my own. I could tune out the voluminous static in my own mind and zero in on a plot, a character, a word. Before my father got sick, I did this because I loved to. After he got sick, the reasons became more complicated.

He was sick for a long time and it has been a long time since he died, and I have spent the last decades of my life being married, having children, writing books, and trying to go back to the years when my father was losing his mind and figure out how I got through them without throwing myself off a roof. What I did wrong (too much to put in one book). What I did right (writing him letters several times a week was right—I know this because even if he couldn't read them, he kept them carefully stowed away in a drawer near his bed as if they were precious things that he really didn't want to lose track of). What I wish I could redo: nothing/everything. And in the process, I have become increasingly unable to disentangle him from his disease. He had lived, after all, for fifty or so years (I'm not sure when the first symptoms appeared, but I'm sure I don't know the half of it because my mother didn't want to tell me) before that, and I had known him for close to a quarter of a century when his mind was intact, before it started to come apart at the seams.

Has literature given me the tools to climb over the wall of a disease that kills memory, not only of the sick person but, in my case, the well one who looked on—to get to the time before the past that I have for a long while defined as starting when my father was diagnosed? Can I get to the other side of that anguished past in order to remember just what I loved so much about him? After all, the depth of love that I have (had) for my father, and the sadness that comes from losing him, can be captured fully only if I can retrieve my healthy father. To make you, the reader, know who he was before he was sick. I shall try to do that now. Can I do here what I love fiction for doing? Create for you, the reader, my father, or more precisely, recreate my memories of him? It should be easier than what novelists do. My dad was real. I'm not creating someone and memories of them *ex nihilo*. At the end of Walt Whitman's poem "Song of Myself," which appeared in the 1855 edition of *Leaves of Grass* (he would revise *Leaves of Grass* until his death in 1892), he writes this:

> Failing to fetch me at first, keep encouraged;
> Missing me one place, search another;
> I stop somewhere, waiting for you.

I read these words and hear my father calling me, urging me to "keep encouraged," coaxing me to continue the "search," reminding me that he stopped (a long time ago), and I should too because he is "waiting" for me. In my mind, he is not angry for "failing to fetch" him. He understands that I couldn't even try, that it's taken me thirty years to try.

The problem is that a wall went up when my dad got Alzheimer's disease. Or I put up a wall, I'm not sure which. But it blocked my view of him. My memories of him when he was healthy started to fade: that he jogged three miles every day in Verona Park, proudly wore pale blue leisure suits, tickled me when he came home from work, took me to Welsh Farms for ice cream on the weekends, was impatient with me for grinding the gears on the stick shift car when he was teaching me how to drive. It hurt so much to remember my father before he got sick that psychically it made some weird kind of sense to forget that he ever was healthy.

I would like to try to climb up and look over that wall now and get at some more of those memories so you will know Jerry Weinstein, born March 16, 1927, died August 12, 1997, but the fact is I've always been a lousy climber. My upper body strength has never been good. In P.E. class at F. N. Brown Elementary School, when the other kids were able to climb the rope up to the gym ceiling, holding on tight and wriggling their bodies to the top, I watched them, alternating between envy and hope (maybe this time I could do it), and then tried to imitate them and always failed. A longstanding inability to do the hula hoop stems from the same bodily weakness. I am pretty sure, though, that my upper mind strength is in good enough shape—at least right now—and I am finally ready to climb to the top and peer over into a different past than the one where my father is losing his mind. Maybe it won't hurt so much now. And even if it does, maybe I'm strong enough to bear it. So let me try to get to where my healthy, loving dad is.

• •

I don't know if he tried to be a great dad or if it just came naturally, but he managed to do what I as a parent have strived to achieve: to be the parent your children would choose. I wrote about that idea in a book about how families were represented in nineteenth-century American literature. I discovered that the families that were put together based on choice were more satisfying than the family one was born into. In novel after novel, children had to find new parents because theirs were usually dead by chapter two (this was the nineteenth century, after all, and people's lifespans were significantly shorter, which clearly has some plusses in that the likelihood of you dying before you get Alzheimer's was higher). The adults who managed to stay alive in the world of the novel took in others' children, if those children didn't succumb to diseases for which medicine wasn't available. In an ironic twist, substitute parents were often better than the real thing. Being released from the bonds of biology allowed people to become their best selves. Now, I certainly didn't want to die (nor did my husband) to liberate my children like in these novels, but I tried to do what I thought was the next best thing. I would imagine myself in a maternal lineup and do everything I could to love my children in the right ways (giving them space; not giving them space; loving them for who they are; encouraging them to be the best person they could be) so that they would say, "I'll take that one."

I totally would have said that about my dad. Here are some things I, an unreconstructed daddy's girl trained in the ways of deconstruction, remember most vividly about my father. It's sort of chronological, but not quite, because the list I offer as evidence of my father's wonderfulness is in the stream of consciousness form favored by novelists such as Virginia Woolf, James Joyce, and of course William Faulkner. Poets use it too. The famous beat poet Allen Ginsberg wrote a poem in 1955 in Berkeley called "A Supermarket in California." He is thinking of his nineteenth-century poetic predecessor and muse, Walt Whitman. In the poem, Ginsberg conjures Whitman's presence and hears him asking these questions of the grocery boys: "Who killed the pork chops? What price bananas? / Are you my Angel?" That's a small taste of stream of consciousness. Whitman's poetry is full of streams that go on and on. Literary critics have called these streams "catalogs," a term derived from the Homeric catalog of ships in Book II of Homer's *Iliad*, which comprises two hundred fifty lines of poetry listing the names of the Greek ships and their leaders that are about to engage in war with Troy. In the poem "Song of Myself," Whitman famously includes catalogs of things, people, experiences, and visions. Here's my catalog for Dad.

He smelled of Old Spice. His favorite alcoholic drink was vodka with grapefruit juice. He loved coffee cake. When people asked him his name, he would always say, "Jerald, with a J, not a G." He was a really good whistler. On Monday nights, I would go to the bank with Dad. He had these accounts called Christmas clubs, which I never really understood because we didn't celebrate Christmas. Sometimes I got lucky, and we got

```
                                    2/22/84

    Dear Cindy,

    Received your letter yesterday and I am
    going to donate the check you sent me to
    your account. It really touched me and made
    me feel very fortunate to have a child as
    good as you who respect what there parents
    did for them over the years.

    Please use  use the money and buy something
    for yourself.

    Thank you for the person that you are.

    All my love
         Dad
```

Letter from Jerry to Cindy dated February 22, 1984

to do my favorite thing at the bank, which was entering the vault. The woman in charge of the vault would open it and there would be rows and rows of narrow drawers, each containing someone's special possessions. Dad would have a small key to our drawer and the woman would have another key, and both keys would open the drawer that belonged to our family. A long rectangular box would be removed, and Dad would look through it. I didn't say anything, just watched. The hush of the place and Dad's seriousness as he went through the papers lead me to believe that this was all really important, and silence was the appropriate response.

As a little girl, I loved sitting in his lap in his big red leather chair watching sports, movies, the television show *The FBI*, hell even *60 Minutes*. For some strange reason, I vividly remember one part of one *FBI* episode. The bad guys cut the telephone cord on the outside of the house, and the people inside were trapped and couldn't call the cops (obviously, this was decades before cell phones). I can't recall how Efrem Zimbalist Jr., the show's lead detective, rescued them, and throughout my childhood I would imagine the phone connection being cut off and having to hide in the dryer, where the bad guys hopefully wouldn't find me. I remember wishing I could remember how the FBI saved the family because not remembering that last part meant potential death by dryer.

Dad would listen to me practice on the piano and if I hit a wrong note, he would say, "Wrong," as if I didn't realize I had made a mistake. Dad would sometimes ask to see my writing assignments. I have a memory of the two of us sitting on the ugly green couch in our living room with him going over one of my essays, written in junior high school for an English class, and reading a sentence out loud. The exact sentence is of course gone from my memory, but the structure of the sentence, the mistake I made, and Dad's correction have stayed with me: "Cindy, a girl from Verona, New Jersey, she had a French poodle named Tocca." To which my dad commented, his voice foreshadowing the red pen I would use in later years to correct student papers, "There is no 'she.'" That's it. I'm pretty sure I never made that mistake again.

Dad was tough on all of us. In an unusual nod to conformity, he decided one day that I should eat peanut butter and jelly sandwiches like every other American kid born in 1960. This, despite the fact that he didn't like them, and I didn't either. I remember sitting at the table in front of the sandwich (on spongy white bread of course), nibbling at the edges and staring at the clock. About an hour later, Dad came into the kitchen, saw that he was not going to win this one, and conceded defeat. He also got it in his head that we should eat the dreaded lima beans that came in the frozen package of vegetables that Mom put in the beef stew. The results tracked with the peanut butter and jelly. There's a funny story about Dad teaching my brother in the early 1970s how to parallel park when knowing how to parallel park was a requirement to get a driver's license. The DMV set the cones at twenty-five feet apart (I think that's the right number), but Dad decided to shave off a few feet, which made it harder for my brother to get the hang of it, but easier to pass that part of the test once he had. I remember my brother coming home, license in hand, commenting on how easy the parallel parking part of the test was and then learning that Dad had purposely put the cones closer together. Dad had high expectations, but really, he only wanted me and everyone he loved to be happy. When I was an adolescent and unhappy, he would ask me, "Why don't you smile anymore?" I didn't really know.

Here's more. When my sister and brother got concert tickets to Sly and the Family Stone, he instructed them to get him one too. He didn't want them to be in Madison Square Garden listening to "I Want to Take You Higher" without being present to somehow ward off incoming dangers—aromatic or otherwise. The way they told it, all of the concertgoers with the exception of my father were standing and screaming to the music, while Dad sat quietly on guard. He liked "Let It Be," up until the part when John starts screaming. In the '60s, at the same time that he started telling people he opposed the Vietnam War, he let his hair grow out, which he had worn in the crew-cut style since serving in the navy during World War II. He took many vitamins and supplements, stopped eating red meat after reading an article on the use of antibiotics in cattle, and ran three miles in Verona Park every day. He learned how to drive a stick shift when his grade school friend, Hatzi (pronounced Hotsy), told Dad to get in the car and drive. He smoked a lot when he was young, started coughing blood, and quit the habit by throwing his last pack of cigarettes out the car window. Frank Sinatra was his favorite singer. He didn't like Bing Crosby (I think this may have had something to do with "White Christmas"). He didn't like when Mom and Grandma Sarah would be on the phone, and they would suddenly start speaking Yiddish. He felt left out. He loved Humphrey Bogart and James Cagney movies. Sophia Loren was his idea of the perfect woman. He hated fakers.

He went to the same school as Philip Roth—Weequahic High School, in Newark—which didn't mean much to me until I read Roth and understood more viscerally my dad's experience of anti-Semitism, race, and my parents' distrust of Roth, which was not uncommon among Jewish families who felt betrayed by Roth's stereotypical depiction of them. When Roth died in 2018, an article appeared with the title "Why Philip Roth Pissed Off So Many Jewish Readers." And in a real-life scene from the Weinstein household that might well have appeared in a Roth novel, my brother was "caught" reading *Portnoy's Complaint* and told to stop reading it immediately. By the way, I haven't been able to finish this novel, because how many scenes of a masturbating adolescent boy can a girl read?

Dad and I went to Knicks games together. I remember going to Madison Square Garden with him in the 1970s and eating dinner beforehand at a greasy spoon place called the Horn and Hardart. We loved the basketball dream team of Walt Frazier, Earl "The Pearl" Monroe, and Wilt "The Stilt" Chamberlain. We

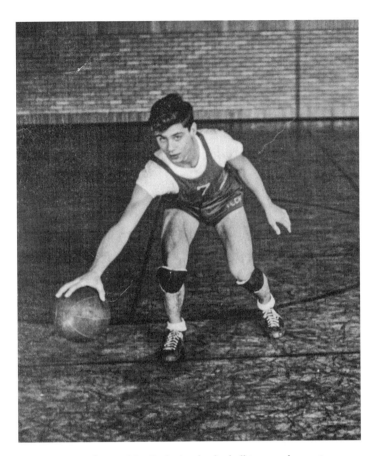

Jerry ("The Machine") playing basketball (year unknown)

made fun of Phil Jackson's "gangly" (that's the word my dad used) arms. Dad would definitely have been surprised that Phil Jackson went on to become a very successful coach of the Los Angeles Lakers (we would have made lots of jokes about how he shouldn't coach his players to play the way he did as a Knick), but by the time that happened, Dad wouldn't know who Phil Jackson was. Although my dad wasn't very tall (5′7″ish), he was a good basketball player in the guard position and his high school coach nicknamed him "The Machine."

He volunteered at the conservative synagogue in town and, when he wasn't stealing the show in the temple's theater productions, his job was to get people to pay their annual dues. The harder people tried to avoid it, the more he dug in. His favorite thing was getting wealthy people who hadn't paid their dues to pony up. One of his special targets was a family that, despite making a lot of money and redoing their kitchen, hadn't sent in a check. When he finally did get the money from them, I remember sitting at the dinner table observing Dad's palpable satisfaction. He was victorious.

He would want me to go with him on Friday nights for Shabbat services, and so there was the perennial choice—do I miss *Get Smart* or go with Dad to temple? It was a tough call, but I'd usually end up going. I remember being at temple once with my dad, and my pop was going to meet us there. Pop showed up in the row behind us, and when I turned around and asked him in a whisper how he was doing (the service had already begun, so the place was quiet, except for the davening—the rocking back and forth in not-so-silent prayer—of the congregants)— he loudly replied, "M-O-K!" Now "M-O-K," for those too young to know, was an advertisement for milk of magnesia, a laxative. In the 1967 commercial, "M-O-K" was code for—you had taken a good shit. I thought Dad and I were going to lose it right then and there.

My dad worked incredibly hard. When I was little, he went to the office six days a week, and then as Apex Electrical Supply took off, the business he owned with my mother's brother, he worked five days a week and then four-and-a-half so he could golf on Friday afternoons. I used to love going with him to the office and typing on the wide-girthed Selectric typewriter or answering the phone, "Apex Electrical Supply, may I help you?" Best of all, though, was getting to ride in the grimy van with him when he was delivering cables, wires, whatever. In those days, there weren't minivans or SUVs, so being in an elevated seat high up on the road counted as a novel experience, as fun. He liked to bowl and dance. His bowling day was Thursday; my mom's Monday. They liked to go dancing at the Meadowbrook Ballroom in Cedar Grove, the town next to Verona. At every bar or bat mitzvah, he would try to teach me how to dance. He liked Robert Goulet, who starred in a 1960s Broadway show called *The Fantastiks* and sang Dad's favorite song, which was "Try to Remember." Talk about foreshadowing. He also loved Cat Stevens's album *Tea for the Tillerman* and Roberta Flack's "The First Time Ever I Saw Your Face." He wasn't materialistic, but he loved his Movado watch, a birthday present from my mother—no numbers, black face, and a diamond where the 12 would have been.

He used to tell me I was afraid of my own shadow, and he was right. Drying to death in a Maytag machine wasn't the only example. Here's a list: the dark, clowns, dolls coming to life (a *Twilight Zone* episode that I saw in Florida that scared the shit out of me for life), the Wicked Witch of the West (her skin, her laugh, the monkeys), my third-grade teacher, who was mean and sent me home from school because she said the gray and beige checked hot pants I was wearing, which my mother had bought me as a birthday present, were too short. The first time I saw my nana without her dentures (I didn't know she wore dentures) terrified me. Her face was disfigured, wizened, collapsed in on itself. Speaking of teeth, I recall my father going to the dentist and consistently refusing Novocaine. The dentist would try to change my dad's mind by telling him how much the procedure was going to hurt, but Dad wouldn't be swayed. I don't think it was entirely about being macho, though he definitely relished narrating the pain and the sound of the drill all while not under the influence. He would say that he preferred the pain to the numbness.

Here's more. He had an aqua Dodge Dart, and he loved it because it lasted forever. Years later, he bought a Dodge Swinger (brown body, cream-colored roof) and hated it. That's when I first learned that the word "lemon" could be applied to cars. He also hated raisins, which upset my Grandma Sarah because she liked to make rugelach, a bite-sized Jewish dessert, with them. He loved Grandma Sarah so much that when he went on a golfing vacation with some of his friends to Bermuda, he took time out of the short trip to visit her in Miami. I remember him saying how happy he was that he had done this because it was the last time he saw her before she died. Dad was like this—he took care of people. He made sure my brother knew how much he was loved even while he was becoming a Buddhist. He made sure that my sister got a dog after my uncle retracted on a promise to give her one from his friend's litter. I think he bought Tocca and brought him home the day of my uncle's betrayal or the next. The first time I saw my father cry was when he came home from the veterinarian having put down Tocca, our beloved dog of thirteen years. I don't think I ever saw him cry about having Alzheimer's, at least I don't remember. But maybe I'm blocking it out. He loved my mother so much that when he got sick, she loved him back with all she had. And he loved me in ways big and small, in ways that make it necessary for me to write this book for him.

I loved to pretend-shave with my dad. He would shake the shaving cream can and put some of it in my palm, which I would then put on my face. We'd laugh. Of course, my razor didn't have a blade in it. For one of Dad's birthdays (I can't remember which one), I found a framed photograph of a daughter and father looking in the mirror, both with shaving cream all over their faces. The caption said, "I remember standing in front of the mirror shaving with my father." My dad's fortieth birthday was great fun. We planned a surprise party, and my very important role was to go out for dinner with Dad, and while we were gone, the guests would come to the house and hide in the living room upstairs. Being nine years old, I could barely contain my excitement, but managed not to blow it. We finished dinner, and he pulled the car into the garage. I was giddy with anticipation. We entered the house through the downstairs (it was a split level) and Dad, as usual, hung his jacket in the hall closet, whereupon he spotted a coat he didn't recognize (it belonged to the mother of a good friend of mine). He wouldn't tell us until the party was over that he saw the coat and immediately realized that something was up. He dutifully acted surprised because he didn't want to disappoint us. This was a Tuesday night.

I know the day of the week because one of the things I remember best is Tuesday nights. Turns out, I was also born on a Tuesday, which of course I don't remember, but Mrs. Weiler in second grade insisted that we find out from our parents on what day of the week we were born because she was teaching us a nursery rhyme, whose first line was, "Monday's child is fair of face." The second line went, "Tuesday's child is full of grace." I remember not really knowing what that meant but liked the sound and the idea of being full of grace. It seemed better than "fair of face" and was obviously way better than Wednesday's child who was "full of woe." I didn't know the words "predictive" or "foreshadowing," but something in me understood that this "grace" thing was something to aim and hope for. Mrs. Weiler also read to us *From the Mixed-Up Files of Mrs. Basil E. Frankweiler* (maybe she was drawn to it because of its echo with her last name), which I loved. Getting stuck in the Metropolitan Museum of Art sounded like so much fun. Mrs. Weiler was also the teacher who made the following bet with the class: come up with a word with a Q that doesn't have a U after it and I'll give you a quarter. It wasn't the quarter that drew me in, but the conundrum posed by the letter Q. Was there a word where Q goes rogue? After many days and dictionary searches, I came up with the word "Iraq." She weaseled out of paying me the quarter by saying Iraq wasn't a common noun, and though I reminded her that she hadn't excluded proper names, I didn't care about the money. I had found the word.

But more important than all this is that Tuesday was the day that Mom went to the YWHA (Young Women's Hebrew Association) and Dad took us out for dinner. This is why we had his surprise birthday party on a Tuesday. Nothing would seem amiss. While Mom spent her Tuesday afternoons getting a massage and *shvitzing* in the sauna and steam rooms, Dad was hanging out with the kids. At first, there were four of us: Dad, Linda, Lyle, and I. Then when Linda went to college, there were three. Then Lyle left for college, and it was Dad and I. There were six years of Tuesdays with just Dad and me.

When it was the four of us, we usually went to this family restaurant called Don's, in Livingston. The booths were roomy, the hamburgers juicy, and the fried chicken crunchy. There was always a wait, about which we would always complain despite knowing there would be a wait. This was our tradition (cue Zero Mostel in *Fiddler on the Roof*): go to Don's, hope there wouldn't be a line, shake our heads about the length of the line, give our name to the hostess, complain about the wait, decide that the food was worth it, and then do it all over again the next week. It occurs to me now that what often broke up the wait was that Dad always seemed to know someone who was in the crowd. It was almost a point of pride that we would go to Don's or anywhere else for that matter and he would have a connection. I guess in today's parlance, we would call it "working the room," but Dad didn't need to work it. He was a natural. As a little girl, I remember thinking that my dad knew everyone and, like me, they loved him. He exuded confidence and warmth.

But the thing I remember most about Don's, besides the food and the perennial wait, was when the wallpaper changed. We walked into Don's one Tuesday night and saw that the walls, which before were nondescript (so much so that I can't remember what they were before the enormity of the transformation that I am about to describe), were suddenly covered with the word "Don's" written all over in red letters on a white background. The word "Don's" was horizontal, vertical, upside down, right side up. Everywhere the eye turned, there was "Don's." It was ridiculous, we thought, because everyone knew they were in Don's, so why do that? We continued to love the food and go there and wait in line and kvetch about it but also wondered if Don's success had gone to his head. Had he become a narcissistic twit, needing to remind everyone that this was his restaurant? We didn't know—until we did—that a part of our tradition at Don's involved not having to engage so intensely with the walls.

I think this attack on tradition that took the form of visually assaulting, name-blaring wallpaper may have had something to do with our decision to try Gary's, in West Orange. This was also around the time Linda went to college, and though Lyle occasionally came to dinner with me and Dad on Tuesday nights, the writing on the wall was clear. Tuesday evenings would soon be just me and Dad. Gary's was no Don's, and Lyle wasn't having any of it. Gary's, however, was a little closer to home and, with good reason, there usually wasn't a wait (the demands of homework were beginning to get in the way of my Tuesday nights). There was no annoying wallpaper, and it had a small jukebox at every table. For a quarter, you could pick three songs. I liked flipping through the options and pushing the letter and the number (C3 or W8) that would give us "Stand by Me," or "You're so Vain," or "I Heard it through the Grapevine." All songs that I liked and knew that Dad did, too.

Although we tried to make the transition from Don's to Gary's, more often than not, Dad and I threw up our hands and surrendered to the relentless wallpaper and Don's onion rings and coleslaw, which were also excellent. What I would give to remember the specifics of just one conversation with Dad at Don's. There are some hazy remembrances: talking about homework; Dad complaining about things at Apex Electric; hearing him talk about Linda going to law school, but thinking he was saying "loss school." I remember thinking, what the heck is loss school? Anyway, truth be told, one exchange does come to mind, but I wish it didn't. This particular conversation I am about to relate concluded many of our dinners at Don's. I dreaded it (I think this is why the content of our dinner conversations remains fuzzy), and it made me unhappy.

A prefatory remark that might seem at first like a non sequitur, considering the previous focus on fried foods and wallpaper, is in order. Math was never my strong suit. It was Dad's, though, and that's one of the reasons the temple leadership put him in charge of collecting dues. Whereas he could easily do math in his head, I needed to write down the problem and even then, the chances of successful completion were slim. Ninth grade was particularly tough when I found myself taking geometry and trying to understand rhombuses. The only thing about rhombuses that interested me was that the word began with "rh." As a result of this unusual combination of consonants, my mind was occupied with coming up with more "rh" words, other than the obvious "rhythm." But that really wasn't the point. My brother was very good at math and he valiantly tried to help. I pretended to understand his instructions, but when he left the room, I found myself drawing larger and larger rhombuses, thinking that if the picture were big enough, I would understand the angles better. Reams of rhombuses covered the bedroom carpet.

Well before rhombuses entered my consciousness, there were word problems. Word problems posed an extreme degree of difficulty, kind of like the gymnast's version of doing a back-flip on the balance beam. I regarded them as a personal affront. Even at a young age, I bristled at the idea of turning words into equations. Calculating the arrival time at a particular destination with two trains traveling at different rates of speed was not fun. What was fun was reading about Jamie and Claudia, in *From the Mixed-Up Files of Mrs. Basil E. Frankweiler*, who were going to take the train from Greenwich, Connecticut, to New York City: "Full fare, one way costs one dollar and sixty cents. Claudia and Jamie could each travel for half of that since she was one month under twelve, and Jamie was well under twelve—being only nine." Now that was math I could get into.

Anyway, all of this throat clearing has to do with what happened when the waitress at Don's left the bill on the table. I can't recall in what grade percentages were first introduced, but my father decided that he would enrich my learning that year by getting me to calculate the tip. The numbers were never even, of course, and that made the calculation harder. Dad would try and make the problem easier by rounding off the numbers, and in a tone of faux patience that conveyed his disappointment in my math abilities, he would say, "If 10 percent of $20 is $2, how much is 15 percent?" I knew the answer but could feel my mind freeze and my tongue thicken and my palms sweat. God, I hated letting him down. Unlike the grammar mistake he pointed out to me on the ugly green sofa, which I would never make again, the lessons in percentages didn't take.

I don't want to end this catalog with a story about math, but instead with two stories about laughter, both of which take place in Florida. Because most of my memories of Florida are grief-laden, these two probably stand out because they are not. The action takes place in our condominium in Fort Lauderdale, where our family is on vacation. Mom is the protagonist in the first with Dad in the background. Dad in the second with Mom in the wings. In the first, I am young, but old enough to have handled on my own the situation which I am about to relate. I did not, however. For some crazy reason that escapes me, my glasses fell in the toilet. I screamed. Mom, without a moment's hesitation, ran into the bathroom, saw the threat, plunged her hand into the toilet with glasses in hand. My reaction was so absurd, and Mom didn't miss a beat, coming to the rescue as if something catastrophic had happened. My brother, sister, and Dad laughed hysterically.

The second story also takes place in the condominium. There are ants. We have been told to eat only in the kitchen so the ants don't follow the food into other rooms. It's late at night. My brother, sister, and I are watching television in the den, and we think that Mom and Dad have fallen asleep. But Dad has not, and he senses that his children are up to no good. He enters the den only to discover that we have snuck some food out of the kitchen. He sternly reprimands us for not listening, turns around, and lo and behold, his pajama bottoms are ripped in the back at the seam and his left cheek, that is, his tush, is exposed. My brother, sister, and I completely lose it, Dad realizes something is up, we try to tell him what's going on in between our hysterics, he finally understands, and dissolves into laughter with us.

This is the person I lost.

A Tragic Juxtaposition

Loss of memory is a hallmark of Alzheimer's disease, and Cindy's "In Memoriam" section is a tribute to a father who could no longer remember. The process of caregiving, brutal and often all-consuming, led Cindy to bury many of the good memories of her father,

Jerry. She notes that writing "In Memoriam" is part of her healing, a healing that takes place decades after her father's death. This conscious act of trying to remember conjures up a flood of buried recollections of her father. Cindy recalls a moral and kind father with charming idiosyncrasies and shapes a beautiful tribute to a remarkable man.

Simultaneously, this chapter offers a window into Cindy's brain, a brain which is highly enriched by the wide range of books she has read and subsequently absorbed into her consciousness and worldview. Books that have influenced Cindy come from a diverse set of authors, ranging from Homer, Charles Dickens, Eugène Ionesco (Cindy, I read *Rhinoceros*, too!), Erich Segal, J. D. Salinger, Albert Camus, J. R. R. Tolkien, and Sinclair Lewis. While Jerry Weinstein's memories were regressing—"This is a mind made blank over time"— Cindy was in graduate school voraciously absorbing book after book and developing new skills as a critic, teacher, and writer. It is a tragic juxtaposition of one brain learning, remembering, and growing, and another that is being decimated by Alzheimer's disease.

Through the use of metaphor, Cindy notes that her father's Alzheimer's disease led to a slow but continuous erasing of the content in his brain—words, events, equations, eventually everything. Cindy imagines his adult mind as a chalkboard that is steadily stripped of content, becoming the blank tablet that he started with: "My dad's mind was like a chalkboard (or whiteboard) filled with equations and words—memories—and Alzheimer's came along and took an eraser to each number, each word. . . . And as if that weren't grotesque enough, the disease had a nasty habit of screwing with the numbers and the words before sending them into oblivion." This chalkboard analogy captures many of the principles that modern neuroscientists have determined about the process of memory— recent, remote, and semantic. While it seems astonishing that Cindy's metaphor is so precise, conjured up without formal training in the science of memory, I have learned that some writers can capture neuroscientific principles more precisely than the scientists who make the basic discoveries.

There is no aspect of cognition that has been more intensely studied than memory, and the picture of how humans remember is continuously being refined. Still, when we try to understand the steps in remembering that have gone awry, we are left with phenomenology that correlates with specific regions in the brain. How we transition from one part of the memory process to the next is still poorly understood, and a comprehensive understanding of human memory is still lacking. With these caveats in mind, in the next paragraphs I describe how a neuroscientist and behavioral neurologist sees and assesses memory. Strap yourselves in, this is not baby stuff.

Overview

Memories are laid down in a stepwise fashion. Remembering begins with an experience, a word, a fact, a number, a song that we encounter activates whatever part of the cerebral cortex that is needed to perceive the input. If we decide to hold that information for longer, the prefrontal cortex becomes active. This is coined working memory. Simultaneously, the hippocampus becomes involved and binds the entire experience to a small number of hippocampal cells. We call this process "encoding." If the experience or word or fact is repeated in an effort to retain the information (we call this consolidation), it is more likely to remain, allowing it to be recalled at a later time. Two factors influence whether or not we remember: the intensity of the stimulus and the effort that we put into re-experiencing or consolidating the event. Finally, after a period of time, some memories become strongly ingrained. The term that we use for these long-held memories is remote memories. Remote memories can be an experience, which is called an episodic memory, or a fact, which we call a semantic memory.

Working Memory

Remembering an experience activates sets of neurons across the brain in a unique pattern that is specific to the experience. This activation depends upon the sensory systems that we use to capture what has happened, whether auditory, visual, olfactory, tactile, or some combination of these senses. Subsequently, a wide variety of factors determines whether the experience will be bound to the complex memory apparatus in the brain so that it can be remembered. For the first moments of remembering (up to thirty seconds), we rely upon our frontal lobes to hold information in the brain. If we decide to remember consciously (or possibly unconsciously) the vision of a flying crow, a list of words, a kiss, a scene from a conversation with a friend, a movie, or a painting in a museum, our frontal lobes go to work and hold that information long enough so that the hippocampus can begin the process of making a more permanent memory. This active effort is called working memory, emphasizing the work, often conscious, that goes into holding information long enough for it to become a permanent memory.

When we test working memory in the clinic, we typically ask a person to remember a list of numbers backward. We start with an easy example. For instance, "Please say these numbers backward: 381." The right answer is "183." We steadily increase the numbers that are to be repeated backward. Most of us remember at least five numbers backward, some of us many more. This process of working memory is relatively normal with Alzheimer's disease, at least in the early stages of the illness.

Episodic Memory: Encoding and Consolidation

The next stage is laying down an episodic memory, the term that is used to describe our ability to remember what, where, and when an experience happened. The fact that we can constantly learn and

lay down new episodes is a fundamental feature of normal existence, and it allows us to learn and grow intellectually. Episodic
memory depends upon a small structure deep in the temporal lobe,
the hippocampus, which permits us to capture and recall later specific memories and experiences.

An example—as I write this paragraph, the time is 6:01 on Monday morning, and a new week of work will soon start. The house
is eerily quiet, except for a slight buzz from the electricity. Today, I
was awakened at 5:15, early for me, by the itching of my nose which
I rubbed with my right hand. The itching disappeared. After getting
up, I peered through the open door into my son's room, where he
leaned over the computer, almost as if in prayer. "Hi Elliot—you're
up early." A nod and a, "Yeah." A brief review of Google News on
my iPhone reveals that the president has attacked four congress-
women in the Democratic Party. I search for the American League
baseball standings, and my Oakland Athletics have won eight of
their last ten games and are steadily moving up the standings. I feel
a little excitement and know that a run for the World Series is possible. Ready for coffee, I walk down the stairs from my bedroom to
the kitchen, put water into the pot, wait for it to boil, pour the hot
water into my French press system, which has ground Philz coffee
at the bottom, placed there the night before. I press down, wait for
four minutes and then pour a large cup of coffee. Instantly ener-
gized by the first sips, I sit down at the computer, eager to write. I
am guilty that it has taken so long to start this chapter—it has been
surprisingly hard. Cindy's face appears in my mind, and I smile, remembering her gentle and oh-so-nuanced way of motivating me
for this final push of our book. I begin writing.

These cascades of neuronal activity that I experienced this morning occurred across the expanse of my brain, but it is the hippocampus that binds all of those activities into an event to be remembered
at a later time. Typically, events like the first ones that I experienced
upon awakening are quickly discarded and forgotten forever. No

one can, and no one should, remember every time that they rub their nose, say hello to their son, or make a pot of coffee. Soon after those experiences, including awakening with an itchy nose, I will begin a grueling week of work with much to accomplish. There will be moments that are far more important to remember than every time I itch. So, the brain is organized not only to help us remember, but there are also systems in place that allow us to forget experiences that are trivial and not necessary for our survival.

As has been noted, the more we relive or practice a prior experience (consolidate), the more likely it is that it will be recalled at a later date. If we don't reexperience a memory over and over again while awake or during sleep, we are likely to forget it. Scientists use the term "consolidation" for the process by which we repeatedly relive an experience to make the binding of the event to the hippocampus stronger. This is what we do when we prepare for a play or an exam, or we try to learn a route in a new neighborhood.

Increasingly, it is evident that sleep is an important factor in the process of consolidation. As we described in our chapter on space, we know that in mice there are individual hippocampal cells that fire while a mouse traverses and learns a maze. During deep sleep, these same exact cells fire again, and scientists suspect that the mouse is reexperiencing travel in that maze, helping to remember where to navigate in the future. So good sleep is important, and if we do things that interfere with deep sleep, we are less likely to consolidate a memory. This topic has become important in Alzheimer's disease, and it is now recognized that deep sleep is a time when we clear bad proteins, like amyloid and tau, from the brain. Some sleeping pills, like benzodiazepines (Valium, Lorazepam), prevent us from getting into deep sleep. Physicians now avoid prescribing them in order to help memory by preventing the aggregation of bad proteins in the brain.

Without a hippocampus, there is only an experience, fleeting, brief, and quickly forgotten. That is what happens to someone with

Alzheimer's disease. It is as if there is a slow release of a toxin in the hippocampus that prevents someone from remembering what they are experiencing. Events happen, but they quickly disappear like the steam in a bathroom when we open the door after a shower. If the hippocampus is unable to bind up a memory, we are trapped in the present and quickly forget new conversations, movies, books, speeches, and even important shared experiences. The Alzheimer's patient plaintively repeats what they have said, again, again, and again, because they cannot remember what they previously asked or were told. The question is erased from the chalkboard. Cindy and Jerry end up talking about the past, as shared present moments can no longer be bound for discussion.

When I test episodic memory in the clinic, I begin by asking the patient about something that has happened recently. Typical questions include: "What did you have for lunch before our visit?"; "What did you eat for dinner the night before?"; or "What happened during a recent holiday?" Often, it is surprising to the patient, and sometimes their loved ones, to see how little is recalled by the Alzheimer's patient. For more formal testing, we ask someone to remember a list of three, eight, or even sixteen words after ten minutes. These word-based memory tasks more directly challenge the left hippocampus, while asking someone to remember a design that they have drawn is more correlated with function of the right hippocampus. So even memory is differentially processed depending upon whether the information is visual or verbal.

Flashbulb Memories

The second principle regarding memory is that if an event is experienced with intense emotion, it may be remembered forever without the need for active rehearsal—it happens without conscious effort. Intense experiences are more likely to become a remote memory that lasts with us for most of our lifetime, even with Alzheimer's disease. I describe one of my most vivid remote memories, one that has been with me for fifty-seven years.

On November 22, 1963, I was an eighth grader at University High School in Madison, Wisconsin. Our morning French class began with the normal shuffling of papers, and I was just easing into my seat when John Kennedy's assassination was announced over the intercom across the school. Time froze, and I felt a flush of fear and sadness. Some of us whispered, "Oh no." I struggled, nearly in panic, with this unthinkable—"our President." After a minute of silence, our young teacher, with auburn hair, dressed in a beautiful knit suit, looked across the class and said—I still remember the cadence and content of the words—"Soyez brave mes élèves" (Be brave, my students). Her face was serious and grave, but it evoked in me an overwhelming sense of empathy. The room became quiet again, and I felt relief. Things were going to be okay. I was proud to be her *élève*, and she had lifted the class from a sense of despair.

That moment, experienced by many others on November 22, 1963, is called a flashbulb memory—something that we remember vividly throughout our life. Sometimes these are experiences that are shared across the world, like Kennedy's assassination or 9/11. Others are intimate: a first kiss, a setback in school, an accident, any event that is highly personal and evokes emotion—extreme emotion. When this happens, the amygdala activates along with the hippocampus, and certain memories are instantly sealed.

Semantic Memory

The types of semantic memories that we store include many of the things that we learn in school: the sound, spelling, and meaning of words; famous paintings or buildings; geographic or literary facts; and the names and faces of acquaintances, athletes, politicians, actors, or other public figures. This information is strongly associated with the function of the anterior temporal lobes. With a specific subtype of frontotemporal dementia, semantic variant primary progressive aphasia, which begins in the anterior temporal lobes, loss of semantic memories is the first manifestation of the illness. In this remarkable illness, the semantic features of our world blur, and birds look similar to dogs and turtles (see page 67), and the names of actors or singers diminish as words are lost. Unlike Alzheimer's disease, where subtle naming deficits are present and clues help the person remember a word, in the semantic patient, even saying a word outright will not improve memory for the word. Vocabulary words, going from easy to hard, the names and faces of famous people, and knowledge about geography can be tested.

As has become evident from the more careful evaluation of different dementia syndromes, like semantic variant primary progressive aphasia, loss of episodic memory as seen in Alzheimer's disease may not occur in other dementias. In Lewy body dementia, visual hallucinations may be the first manifestation; in behavioral variant FTD, it is behavior change, not memory loss, that happens first; and with semantic variant, the inability to recognize words or faces may happen first. Even with Alzheimer's disease, the first manifestation of the illness is not always a deficit in episodic memory. The first symptom can be language, executive, or visuospatial dysfunction.

Imperfections in Current Models of Memory

Many mysteries still remain regarding how humans retain memories over time. It is hard to test remote memory, and there are no standards because we all carry remote memories that are unique to us. Therefore, we are never certain about what experiences or knowledge an individual previously possessed. Every study on remote memory has to be carefully planned and validated based upon relative certainty regarding the memories that the subject has. Compared to the massive literature on episodic memory, there is still a paucity of papers on how recent memories become remote or lost.

In one remarkable study by Edmond Teng and Larry Squires called "Memory for Places Learned Long Ago Is Intact after Hippocampal Damage," the authors studied a man with severe bilateral hippocampal damage who had no ability to remember new events. After multiple home visits with extensive testing and interaction, the subject treated Drs. Teng and Squires as if they had never met before. Yet, he could remember maps of Castro Valley, where he had lived as a young boy, as well as or better than classmates with whom he was together when he was seven. The authors concluded that spatial maps aren't permanently stored in the hippocampus. Rather, the hippocampus and related structures in the temporal lobe were needed to learn (or form) spatial and nonspatial information, but very remote memories eventually became independent of the hippocampus. We still don't know what, when, and why memories become hippocampal independent.

Cognitive Reserve

The importance of education early in life as a way to protect ourselves from memory loss in old age supports the concept of cognitive reserve. That is, some of us are protected from neurodegenerative disorders based upon the way that our brains develop across the lifetime. Yaakov Stern, a neuropsychologist at Columbia School of Medicine, pioneered studies on how we obtain cognitive reserve. Research across many cultures, countries, and languages now suggests that people with a high level of education are more resistant to the Alzheimer's process than people with low education. What this means is that in someone who is literate, with more than a high school level education, there needs to be a higher burden of amyloid and tau in the brain before symptoms of cognitive difficulties emerge, compared to someone who is illiterate, where a much lower burden of pathology will cause symptoms. It appears that even though the disease is present in the brain, education protects us until the burden becomes overwhelming. Living in an intellectually stimulating environment is good for our brain health and makes us less vulnerable, more resilient to the effects of insults, whether they are stroke, trauma, Alzheimer's disease, or frontotemporal dementia.

What is it about education, intellectual curiosity, and taking on cognitive challenges that protects our brain? The current hypothesis is that a lifetime of intellectual activity increases the number of connections, or synapses, in the brain, changing the threshold for when an insult will cause cognitive impairment. These synapses grow when we learn and are responsible for the brain's cognitive activity. Supporting this idea have been new and pioneering studies by neurologist Elisa Resende, described in our chapter on words. Dr. Resende studied cognitively healthy fifty-year-olds in Belo Horizonte, Brazil, who were illiterate and had less than four years of education versus those who went further in school and were able to read. Remarkably, even though the low-education group was cognitively normal at the time of the study, their hippocampi were small compared to the hippocampi in people who went further in school. Did the voracious reading that Cindy and I did as children protect us from Alzheimer's disease later in life? Maybe. Like many other aspects of health, social deprivation, even early in life, predisposes us to a multitude of bad health outcomes throughout our life, including Alzheimer's disease. Now, Dr. Resende is initiating studies that bring reading to her middle-aged illiterate population to see whether it can increase the size of their hippocampi and protect them from Alzheimer's disease.

There are many ongoing studies looking at the effectiveness of cognitive stimulation as a protection strategy or treatment for healthy elders who are cognitively normal, show mild cognitive impairment, or suffer from dementia. The value of stimulating activities, like Sudoku, crossword puzzles, computer games, or online courses is still unknown, and it is possible that simply living a stimulating life enhanced by social engagement and reading is equally protective. We still don't know whether, or what type of, cognitive stimulation is most likely to increase cognitive reserve. Yet, sensible lifestyle approaches based on keeping the mind active and stimulated are now routinely recommended for brain health. Similarly, as is documented in the next section, lack of sleep impairs our ability to retain memories, and may even make it more likely that we develop dementia. Therefore, like the topic of cognitive reserve, improving sleep across the lifetime has become a common focus of dementia prevention and therapy.

Repressed Memories: How the Unconscious Works

Cindy begins the section "In Memoriam" describing her father and notes, "There must be many stories about his past and our shared past that he would have told me if he hadn't gotten sick, and those events died when my father died. I lost the past, too. The past we shared before he lost those things. I'm going to see if I can find it." Her intense engagement in studies, work, family, life left the good memories of her father dormant. But as she writes this book, she recovers with a rush of buried memories, bringing up questions about how we frame the world as it relates to our past and where we store hidden memories.

Like Cindy, all of us carry memories that seem to lie dormant for days, weeks, years, even decades, when suddenly they are consciously recalled. Do memories really sit in the brain, quiescent and untouched until they are consciously reexperienced? Do these memories really lie quiescent for decades? Maybe not, if we extrapolate from the research of basic science colleagues who electrically record the hippocampi of mice and rats while they are learning to navigate a maze. As the rodents navigate a maze, small numbers of cells in the hippocampus discharge every time they move through a specific place. It is as if every place in the maze is represented by a few cells in the hippocampus. During deep sleep, that same pattern of firing occurs, suggesting that the rodent is reexperiencing moments that occurred during the day or previous days while learning the environment of the maze. So sleep is a time for reexperiencing and consolidating memories, even if we are not consciously aware of the memories in the day.

For example, last night I dreamed of walking down a road remembered from my childhood that was flanked on one side by a golf course and the other side by two beautiful blocks of elegant houses that were built in the 1940s. This block contained a flood of memories for me, ranging from visits with friends from ages six to seventeen, being bitten by a dog, playing golf, skipping school, and listening with my friend to the Velvet Underground banana album as a senior in high school. When we are unconscious in deep sleep, floods of memories are being reexperienced, consolidated, and reshaped. In dreams, we take clips of memories from our remote past, integrate recent memories that may be anxiety-producing in the present, review facts or landscapes that we may want to learn, and create a new world that projects us through various scenarios imagined. Most of this happens without any conscious awareness of the dreams, unless, of course, we happen to be awakened before the dream has finished. How do we ever keep track of what is real and what is imagined?

Psychologists like Sigmund Freud wrote extensively about the unconscious state and its strong influence on our daily behavior. For Freud and his disciples, the dream was an inroad to our inner drives, motivations, fears, and hopes. He suspected that we suppressed threatening ideas that we were unwilling to face. What Freud could not have predicted is that dreams and sleep are extremely important for studying mechanisms of memory, not just in humans, but in animals as well. While still unproven, it is easy to postulate that the frequent consolidation and reshaping of memories during deep sleep is one of the ways that we maintain memories across time. If consolidation and reexperiencing happen during deep sleep, it means that during this time, we do not have logical or conscious control of what we remember. Therefore, it is no surprise that many of our memories are distorted, even false. Psychologist Daniel Schacter at Harvard has found that we all carry memories that are inaccurate. With Alzheimer's disease, false memories may become more common, even leading to delusional endorsement of events that never happened, but it is important to realize that memory is fragile, even in the cognitively healthy. The complex processes by which the hippocampus binds, consolidates, and uses old memories to plan future actions lies at the core of this vulnerability.

Cindy's memories of her father are a source of joy and pride for her and should have a sustaining influence upon future generations, beginning with her children. This is the way that societies sustain myth, legend, cultural continuity, and knowledge. Cindy's book transforms the tragedy of Jerry Weinstein's memory loss into knowledge, tribute, and hope, generating new memories for all of us.

Here is my own version of translating memory into a tribute. The picture on the back cover is titled *The Life and Death of Billy Miller*, and it is a watercolor from my mother, Harriet Bernice Sanders Miller, MFA. Mom, soon to be ninety-four, is an artist and art educator who loves children and dogs. This picture is her dedication to an incredible blue merle Australian Shepherd named Billy, who lived with her and my father on the ocean in San Pedro, California. The picture frames, through multiple squares, Billy's life. There are three main themes. The first squares are mystical and present Billy's birth and origins; the second squares show the palm trees that Mom, Dad, and Billy walked by every day during their time together living on the ocean; and the last squares represent Billy's death and his rise into the universe. Thousands and thousands of experiences are abstracted into the frames, which represent a life of a very special dog shared together with my parents. The picture, profoundly beautiful and sad for me, captures the brief moments of our lives, remembered and crystallized into squares.

Afterword

The Brain—is wider than the Sky—
EMILY DICKINSON, 1862

5.8 million Americans live with Alzheimer's disease.
ALZHEIMER'S ASSOCIATION, 2019

We juxtapose Emily Dickinson's poem about the grandeur of the brain with the Alzheimer's Association's staggering statistic about the number of people in America whose brains are suffering from Alzheimer's disease, the most common form of dementia. This is an epidemic of our time, one for which we are poorly prepared individually and as a society. Until a prevention emerges, this book is one small step to help patients, families, and caregivers understand and cope with an illness that always kills the patient and often devastates their loved ones. This book brings together the humanities and the sciences in order to describe that devastation and to chart a path beyond it.

Dickinson's poetry about the brain speaks to what neurologists have known for some time: that the complexities of the brain are "wider than the sky" and "deeper than the sea." When neurons in the brain start dying, imagery shows black spots where brain matter once lived. For Dickinson, the sky darkens and one drowns in the sea. Literature, in this case poetry, harmonizes with the story of the brain that neurologists tell.

This book is the story of Jerry Weinstein as told through our eyes. There are two pairs of eyes: one an English professor's; the other, a neurologist's. We began this book with a vision defined by our disciplines. We would bring to the telling of Jerry's story the perspective of a daughter and her love of literature, with that of a physician and his passion for science. In the course of writing this book, however, our disciplines overlapped, our vocabulary merged, and our vision, which was initially doubled, came into alignment. The magnetic pull of interdisciplinary thinking moved Cindy toward neurology and Bruce toward literature. As Bruce got to know Cindy's father, Cindy got to know his. Our point of departure—what made us click that first time we met in UCSF's Sandler Building when Bruce asked Cindy, "Do you want to learn some science?" and she said, "Yes, and what books do you most enjoy?—was always empathy. Our book is the expression of that empathy. Dementia takes us all on different journeys when it enters our world. Yet we hope that the commonalities of everyone's experience will make this very personal story helpful to the reader.

ACKNOWLEDGMENTS

Cindy

The number of people I have to thank for making this book possible is daunting. Without Jim, none of these pages would have or could have been written. I owe him everything. My love for Sarah and Sam gave me the strength and conviction to write this book. This story of a grandfather they never knew, who would have profoundly loved them (and they him), attempts to capture what it would have been like to have had my father, their grandfather, in their lives. This book is for them.

Dori Hale, reader and friend extraordinaire, helped me get through some of the toughest times recorded here and then the remembering of them. I will forever be in her debt for many reasons, large and small, including the fact that she found me a room of my own in Berkeley in which to write this book. Arlene Zuckerberg, college roommate and empath par excellence, knew me before Dad got sick, during, and after. She has been by my side since I was seventeen. Linda, Lyle, and I went through this together. To Linda, thank you for taking such good care of Mom and Dad during all of those difficult years. To Lyle, thank you for making and keeping the promise to Dad that you would watch over me.

I am so lucky to count Cathy Jurca as a friend and colleague. Not only did she write me a letter of recommendation for UCSF, she is a brilliant and generous person. Bob Levine wrote a second letter of recommendation, and I am grateful to him for his longtime friendship (and passion for Herman Melville's *Pierre*). Many friends and colleagues took time to read chapters of this book. Thanks go to Rachel Adams, John Brewer, Shival Dasu, Marcy Dinius, Melissa Fox, Jane Garrity, Ming Guo, Bruce Hay, Ken Kosik, Mariah Proctor-Tiffany, Nancy Ruttenburg, Julia Stern, Eric Sundquist, and my childhood friend Elise Yousoufian, whose memories of my father were written in her diary entries that she kept and shared with me. Thank you to Lenny Cassuto, Rita Charon, Chris Gabbard, Dehn Gilmore, Sharon Maher, Hiromi and Shizuyo Matsuda, Laura Mazer, Ramona Naddaff, Samuel Otter, Ralph Savarese, Elisa Tamarkin, and Clare Wellnitz for talking to me about the project. Special thanks to Tracy Dennison and Michelle Hawley, whose patience and friendship have spanned many years and countless conversations that have made this book better. Nancy Rhodes has also been an invaluable reader and listener, and I am grateful to her for years of support and consolation. I wish Timo were here so I could thank him again for teaching me how to read Melville and for being my friend.

Caltech has been extraordinary. Tom Rosenbaum, Dave Tirrell, and Jean-Laurent Rosenthal gave me the gift of a year to study neurology at UCSF, to read as many books as possible, and to write this book with Bruce. As if that weren't enough, they invited me to speak about that time at a board of trustees meeting where Sue Woolscy was in the audience, and asked to read chapters of the book and shared them with Barbara Kline Pope, director of Johns Hopkins University Press. I am also grateful to Shirley Malcom, Caltech trustee and friend, who has been a steadfast supporter. Thanks to David Anderson and David Baltimore for helping me figure out how to get to the Memory and Aging Center at UCSF. Thank you to Kaushik Bhattacharya and Stacey Scoville for their help while I was away, and to Peggy Blue, Regina Colombo, Alicia Creger, Helen Duong, Linda Krippner, Avi Leibovici, Cierina Marks, Nancy O'Connor, and Carol Schuil for taking time to provide feedback on chapters.

The UCSF community as a whole, and the GBHI group in particular, has been amazing. Special thanks to the doctors, artists, and professionals in the GBHI cohort: Kirsty Bobrow, Maritza Pintado Caipa, Gabri Christa, Walt Dawson, Stefanie Piña Escudero, Laís Fajersztajn, Agustín Ibañez, Stefania Ilinca, Ophir Keret, Emi Kiyota, Alex Kornhuber, Lingani Mbakile-Mahlanza, Shamiel McFarlane, Maira Okada de Oliveira, Myriam De la Cruz Puebla, Rowena Richie, Yasuhiro Tanaka (honorary GBHI'er), and senior fellows, Eléonore Bayen, Phaedra Bell, Talita Rosa, and Claire Sexton. Big thanks to Suzee Lee, the perfect mentor. Also thank you to the UCSF community (past and present), including Rosalie Gearhart, Leslie Goss, Joel Kramer, Diane Madsen, Maria Luisa Mandelli, Mary De May, Zachary Miller, Eleanor O'Brien, Nicole

Plata, Kate Possin, Salvo Spina, and Stacey Yamamoto. Special thanks to Suzanne Kawahara. Their collective input and generosity helped to secure funding from the Alzheimer's Association and the Alzheimer's Society UK, to which I owe a significant debt of gratitude.

The Johns Hopkins University Press editorial team, Joe Rusko, Adelene Jane Medrano, and Kyle Kretzer, and the Press director, Barbara Kline Pope, have been terrific. Thanks to them and to Caroline Prioleau, for stepping in at a crucial time and helping to make this book a reality.

Last but not least, thank you Bruce. My father and mother would have loved you. You are the doctor he/we didn't get to have. Whatever simple twist of fate led me to you, I will always be grateful.

Bruce

Writing this book with Cindy has been an unexpected gift, allowing me to work with Cindy, a new and dear friend, while opening me up to different ways of thinking about science, my patients, my family, and my own brain. Describing the neuroscience of cognitive impairment to a lay audience frequently sent me back to the scientific literature as I pondered the complex underpinnings of what happened to Cindy and her father as it related to memory, space, language, and behavior. Hearing about Cindy's battle with her father's Alzheimer's disease reminded me that every time someone comes to my office with a cognitive disorder, there is intense fallout that touches upon the patient's wide circle of friends and loved ones.

With my drafts for each chapter, I loved Cindy's gentle manner of prodding me when I ducked the personal and slid to the generic. This book became a unique opportunity to self-reflect and describe my own peculiar journey as a scientist, clinician, son, grandson, father, and grandfather. No one has a life that is easy, but this book helped me to realize how lucky—privileged—I have been, and how that privileged life has made it possible for me to become a behavioral neurologist. While writing, I experienced a flood of gratitude as I thought back to my grandparents' and parents' encouragement of my reading, and my decision to become a physician. Also, I reflected upon how generous my brilliant and beautiful wife, Deborah, has been in allowing me to pursue a career in medicine and science.

My ancestors worked ferociously hard so that I could have the opportunities that came to me. My paternal grandparents, William and Helen Miller's kindness and generosity helped me to become a physician. I lived with them for two years while obtaining a post-baccalaureate degree in chemistry at Butler University on my path to medical school. My mother's parents, Herman and Dorothy Sanders, strongly believed in education, and starting at a young age my evenings reading with Herman were a huge boost for my brain and my confidence. Milton, my father, was a fun-loving and generous academic psychiatrist whose desire to help people, whatever their status in society, was inspiring. I have tried to model that generosity and still miss going to him for advice. Mom, beautiful and stylish with unbounding energy, is a sustaining light for me. No family has ever had a fiercer advocate. Her passions are art, children, animals, and family. During this COVID-19 epidemic I am particularly proud of my grandson Mason (age seven) for his readings to her. My children Hannah and Elliot enrich my life every day, as do Hannah's husband Seth Whitehead and my grandchildren Mason and Addie.

My mentors Jeff Cummings and Frank Benson at UCLA were exemplary in every way. At UCSF, I thank the three hundred people who work at the Memory and Aging Center. They inspire me every day. In particular, Rosalie Gearhart has encouraged my popular writing and has worked with me from the time that I arrived in San Francisco in 1998. Similarly, Caroline Prioleau edits everything I write and is responsible for the figures in this book. Cindy and I came together through the Global Brain Health Institute, and Chris Oechsli, Victor Valcour, Ian Robertson, and Brian Lawlor have all been wonderful colleagues during the founding of this organization. Finally, I dedicate this book to my two friends from medical school, psychiatrist Steve Read, emergency physician Bruce Fleming, and my friend Dan Geschwind, neurologist and geneticist.

GLOSSARY

acetylcholine (chemical, n). A chemical neurotransmitter that helps neurons communicate.

agraphia (Greek, n). The loss or impairment of the ability to write.

alexia (Greek, n). The loss or impairment of the ability to read.

alpha-synuclein (chemical, n). A protein found in the brain and the main component in Lewy bodies and a pathological marker of Parkinson's disease.

Alzheimer's disease (medical, n). A progressive, degenerative neurological disease that typically affects memory and other important mental functions.

amyloid-beta-42 (chemical, n). A protein derived from amyloid precursor protein and made of 42 amino acids.

amyloid plaques (chemical, n). A clump of insoluble amyloid-beta-42 protein that is a pathological marker of Alzheimer's disease.

amyotrophic lateral sclerosis (ALS, or Lou Gehrig's disease) (medical, n). A progressive, degenerative neurological disease that affects nerve cells in the brain and spinal cord that control motor function.

anomia (Greek, n). The loss or impairment of the ability to recall the names of objects.

anosognosia (Greek, n). The lack of awareness or denial of illness that often accompanies neurodegenerative conditions.

aphasia (Greek, n). The loss or impairment of the ability to produce and/or understand language.

atrophy (Greek, n). The breakdown and loss of tissue.

Benson's syndrome. See **posterior cortical atrophy**

biomarker (medical, n). Also called biological marker. An objective measure of a biological state that helps make a diagnosis and measure disease progression.

bildungsroman (German, n). A genre that describes the development of the protagonist in a literary work.

brainstem (medical, n). The back part of the brain at the top of the spinal cord that regulates breathing, heart rate, blood pressure, sleeping, and other essential functions.

broygus (Yiddish, adj). Having a grumpy or sullen demeanor.

bruxism (medical, n). The unconscious grinding, clenching, or gnashing of the teeth.

bubelah (Yiddish, n). A term of endearment meaning sweetie or darling.

cellular inclusion (medical, n). A small entity found within a cell.

cerebral cortex (medical, n). The highly folded, outermost layer of the cerebrum in mammals.

cerebrum (Latin, n). The largest part of the human brain, made up of the two cerebral hemispheres and the cerebral cortex.

chronic traumatic encephalopathy (CTE) (medical, n). A progressive, degenerative neurological disease associated with repeated head trauma.

clinical presentation (medical, n). The physical signs and symptoms associated with an illness that lead to a specific diagnosis.

consolidation (medical, n). The process by which a new memory is converted into stable, long-lasting memory.

dementia with Lewy bodies. See **Lewy body dementia**

disinhibition (medical, n). The inability to stop oneself from engaging in inappropriate social behaviors that appear tactless, rude, or offensive.

encoding (medical, v). The process by which a perception of thought is converted into memory.

episodic memory (medical, n). The memory of a specific personal experience.

ex nihilo (Latin, prep. phrase). Out of nothing, or out of nowhere.

flashbulb memory (medical, n). A vivid, strong memory of a personally significant moment in time.

frontal lobe (medical, n). The front part of each of the cerebral hemispheres, which regulates and mediates higher intellectual functions, such as emotions, cognition, error detection, volition, and a sense of self.

fronto-opercular region (medical, n). An area of cortex tucked underneath the folds of the frontal lobe along the Sylvian fissure, or lateral sulcus (the long crease that separates the temporal lobe from the frontal and parietal lobes).

frontotemporal dementia (FTD) (medical, n). The umbrella term for the clinical syndromes of behavioral variant frontotemporal dementia (bvFTD), semantic variant primary progressive aphasia (svPPA), and nonfluent variant primary progressive aphasia (nfvPPA). All share involvement of the frontal and temporal lobes of the brain. This term sometimes refers specifically to bvFTD.

gyrus, gyri (medical, n). The highly folded pattern of ridges in the cerebral cortex.

H&E stain (hematoxylin and eosin stain) (medical, n). The most widely used tissue stain in medical diagnosis. Hematoxylin stains the cell nuclei blue or dark purple, and eosin stains the cytoplasm pink—combining to provide an overview of the tissue structure. Lewy bodies are eosinophilic and stain pink.

hippocampus (medical, n). A structure found in the temporal lobes, below the cerebral cortex, that is involved in memory.

Jakob-Creutzfeldt disease (medical, n). A rapidly progressive, degenerative neurological disease caused by abnormal prions, which are microscopic infectious agents made of protein.

kaddish (Hebrew, n). A prayer said at Jewish synagogue services, also frequently recited during funerals and during the time of mourning.

kvell (Yiddish, v). To express pride and delight.

kvetch (Yiddish, v). To complain.

Lewy bodies (medical, n). Pathological deposits of the protein alpha-synuclein found within neurons.

Lewy body dementia (medical, n). The Lewy body dementias are progressive, degenerative neurological diseases associated with movement, visual hallucinations, and fluctuations in thinking skills or attention. They are characterized by the presence of Lewy bodies.

logopenic variant primary progressive aphasia (medical, n). A progressive, degenerative neurological disease that affects the temporal lobes and leads to trouble with word finding.

Lou Gehrig's disease. See **amyotrophic lateral sclerosis**

magnetic resonance imaging (MRI) (medical, n). An imaging technique that uses magnetism, radio waves, and a computer to produce noninvasive, high-quality images of internal structures of the body.

metabolism (medical, n). The biochemical process by which materials are turned into energy.

mild cognitive impairment (medical, n). A condition defined by deficits in memory that do not significantly impact daily functioning and may remain stable for years. However, some individuals with MCI develop cognitive deficits and functional impairment consistent with Alzheimer's disease.

neurodegenerative disease (medical, n). A chronic, progressive neurological disease that leads to the loss of brain tissue and function.

neurofibrillary tangles (medical, n). Pathological clusters of the tau protein found within neurons.

nonfluent variant primary progressive aphasia (medical, n). A progressive, degenerative neurological disease that affects the frontal lobes and leads to trouble pronouncing words or increasing difficulty vocalizing words.

occipital lobe (medical, n). The back part of each of the cerebral hemispheres, which helps to process visual information.

oral exam (orals). A spoken, intensive Q&A between PhD candidate and professors in her field, preceding writing of the doctoral thesis.

orthograph (Greek, n). The visual marks, forms, or structures of written language.

parietal lobe (medical, n). The upper sides of each of the cerebral hemispheres, which help to process sensory information and movement.

positron emission tomography (PET) scans (medical, n). An imaging technique that uses a brain camera and radioactive material (a tracer) to produce images of metabolic activity and protein buildup in the brain.

posterior cortical atrophy (Benson's syndrome) (medical, n). A rare, visual variant of Alzheimer's disease.

prodromal stage (medical, n). The time when early symptoms of a disease are mild or appear before the more characteristic disease symptoms occur.

remote memory (medical, n). The long-term storage of information from working memory that can, theoretically, be retrieved indefinitely.

rugelach (Yiddish, n). A buttery, flaky, dense Jewish pastry-cookie, usually filled with chocolate chips, raisins, or nuts.

salience network (medical, n). A large neural network in the frontal and insular parts of the brain; it detects and attends to stimuli of interest.

shlepp (Yiddish, v). To haul or drag an item or oneself with difficulty.

semantic memory (medical, n). The type of memory used for storing factual information and meaning.

semantic variant primary progressive aphasia (medical, n). A progressive, degenerative neurological disease that affects the temporal lobes and leads to trouble understanding the meaning of words, finding words, or naming people and objects.

shiva (Hebrew, n). A ritualistic period of mourning in Judaism, typically lasting for a week. Family members of the lost loved one gather together and are encouraged to grieve through disengaging with the outside world.

shvitz (Yiddish, v). To sweat.

sulcus, sulci (medical, n). The highly folded pattern of furrows in the cerebral cortex.

TAR DNA-binding protein 43 (TDP-43) (medical, n). A protein that controls the production of versions of other proteins; the abnormal TDP-43 clumps are found in several diseases that lead to the clinical syndrome of frontotemporal dementia or ALS.

tau (medical, n). A protein in the body that normally helps form the cellular structure used for cellular transportation.

temporal lobe (medical, n). The lower sides of each of the cerebral hemispheres, which help to process language, emotion, and memory.

tenure. A permanent position earned by a professor.

vascular dementia (medical, n). A progressive, degenerative neurological disease caused by damaged blood vessels, resulting in reduced or blocked blood flow to the brain and leading to symptoms that often look like Alzheimer's disease.

verklempt (Yiddish, adj). To be emotionally overwhelmed, used in a positive or negative context.

working memory (medical, n). The limited-capacity memory that temporarily holds a perception or thought before either forgetting it or moving it into long-term storage.

SUGGESTED READINGS

Benson, Frank, and Jeffrey L. Cummings. *Dementia: A Clinical Approach*. 1992.
Berchtold, Nicole, and Carl Cotman. "Evolution in the Conceptualization of Dementia and Alzheimer's Disease: Greco-Roman Period to the 1960s." *Neurobiology of Aging*. 1998;19:173–89.
Camus, Albert. *The Stranger*. 1942.
Chopin, Kate. *The Awakening*. 1899.
de Saussure, Ferdinand. *Course in General Linguistics*. 1916.
Dickens, Charles. *David Copperfield*. 1850.
Dickens, Charles. *Great Expectations*. 1861.
Dickens, Charles. *Oliver Twist*. 1838.
Dickinson, Emily. "The Brain—is wider than the Sky— ." 1862.
Dickinson, Emily. "I felt a Funeral, in my Brain," 1861.
Dreiser, Theodore. *An American Tragedy*. 1925.
Edwards, Jonathan. "Sinners in the Hands of an Angry God." 1741.
Eliot, T. S. "The Love Song of J. Alfred Prufrock." 1915.
Emerson, Ralph Waldo. "Nature." 1836.
Fariña, Richard. *Been Down So Long It Looks Like Up to Me*. 1966.
Faulkner, William. *The Sound and the Fury*. 1929.
Fielding, Henry. *The History of Tom Jones, a Foundling*. 1749.
Friedan, Betty. *The Feminine Mystique*. 1963.
Ginsberg, Allen. "Kaddish." 1961.
Ginsberg, Allen. "A Supermarket in California." 1955.
Gladwell, Malcolm. "Complexity and the Ten-Thousand-Hour Rule." 2013.
Goedert, Michel. "Oskar Fischer and the Study of Dementia." *Brain*. 2009;132:1102–111.
Golding, William. *Lord of the Flies*. 1954.
Greer, Germaine. *The Female Eunuch*. 1970.
Hawthorne, Nathaniel. *The Scarlet Letter*. 1850.
Homer. *Iliad*.
Hughes, Thomas. *Tom Brown's School Days*. 1872.
Ionesco, Eugène. *Rhinoceros*. 1959.
Irving, Washington. "Rip Van Winkle." 1819.

Ivry, Benjamin. "Why Philip Roth Pissed Off So Many Jewish Readers." *Forward*. 2018.

Joyce, James. *Ulysses*. 1922.

Katzman, Robert. "The Prevalence and Malignancy of Alzheimer's Disease: A Major Killer." *Archives of Neurology*. 1976;33:217–28.

Kerouac, Jack. *On the Road*. 1957.

Konigsburg, E. L. *From the Mixed-Up Files of Mrs. Basil E. Frankweiler*. 1967.

Lewis, Sinclair. *Main Street*. 1920.

Melville, Herman. "Bartleby, the Scrivener." 1853.

Melville, Herman. *Mardi*. 1849.

Melville, Herman. *Moby-Dick*. 1851.

Michener, James. *The Source*. 1965.

Miller, Z. A., M. L. Mandelli, K. P. Rankin, et al., "Handedness and Language Learning Disability Differentially Distribute in Progressive Aphasia Variants." *Brain*. 2013;136:3461–73.

Nabokov, Vladimir. *Lolita*. 1955.

Norris, Frank. *McTeague*. 1899.

Orwell, George. *1984*. 1949.

Pirsig, Robert. *Zen and the Art of Motorcycle Maintenance*. 1974.

Poe, Edgar Allan. *The Narrative of Arthur Gordon Pym*. 1838.

Poe, Edgar Allan. "The Raven." 1845.

Pynchon, Thomas. *Gravity's Rainbow*. 1973.

Pynchon, Thomas. *Inherent Vice*. 2009.

Roth, Philip. *Portnoy's Complaint*. 1969.

Salinger, J. D. *Catcher in the Rye*. 1951.

Segal, Erich. *Love Story*. 1970.

Shakespeare, William. *Hamlet*. 1609.

Stevenson, Robert Louis. *Strange Case of Dr. Jekyll and Mr. Hyde*. 1886.

Stowe, Harriet Beecher. *Uncle Tom's Cabin*. 1852.

Teng, Edmond, and Larry Squires. "Memory for Places Learned Long Ago Is Intact after Hippocampal Damage." *Nature*. 1999;400:675–77.

Thomas, Dylan. "Do Not Go Gentle into That Good Night." 1951.

Thoreau, Henry David. *Walden*. 1854.

Tolkien, J. R. R. *The Hobbit*. 1937.

Tomlinson, Bernard, Gary Blessed, and Martin Roth. "Observations on the Brains of Demented Old People." *Journal of the Neurological Sciences*. 1970;11:205–42.

Tomlinson, Bernard, Gary Blessed, and Martin Roth. "Observations on the Brains of Non-Demented Old People." *Journal of the Neurological Sciences*. 1968;7:331–56.

Turner, Frederick Jackson. "The Significance of the Frontier in American History." 1893.

Twain, Mark. *Adventures of Huckleberry Finn*. 1884.

Uris, Leon. *Exodus*. 1958.

Weinstein, Cindy. *The Literature of Labor and the Labors of Literature: Allegory in Nineteenth-Century American Fiction*. 1995.
Weinstein, Cindy. *Time, Tense, and American Literature: When Is Now?* 2015.
Whitman, Walt. *Leaves of Grass*. 1855.

INDEX

Page numbers in *italics* indicate images or tables